MEDICINAL FARMING

EMPOWERING FARMERS IN INDIA

MEDICINAL **FARMING**

EMPOWERING FARMERS IN INDIA

By

Dr. V.K. Singh, Ph.D.

Project Director & Former Deputy Director (Botany)
CCRUM Headquarters, Ministry of AYUSH,
Government of India, New Delhi – 110023

2025

Medicinal Farming: Empowering Farmers in India
Dr. V.K. Singh, Ph.D.

Cover Page Photographs: Tulsi, Safed Musli, Kanta Karanj, Mushkdana

DISCLAIMER

The information contained in this book is provided for general informational purposes only. While every effort has been made to ensure the accuracy and reliability of the content, the author and publisher make no representations or warranties, expressed or implied, regarding the completeness, accuracy, or suitability of the information for any particular use.

ISBN : 979-8-3304-7745-6

Flames Creations | Design Services Provided by Flames Creations

EMPOWERING FARMERS: ENHANCING LIVELIHOODS

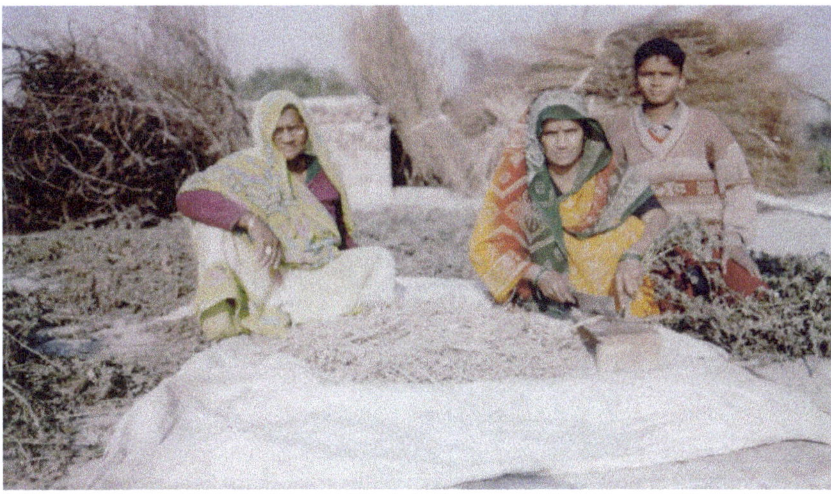

Fig 1: Women farmers in Baragaon Okhlana, Aligarh, processing Ashwagandha roots (Withania somnifera) cultivated in their fields, for marketing.

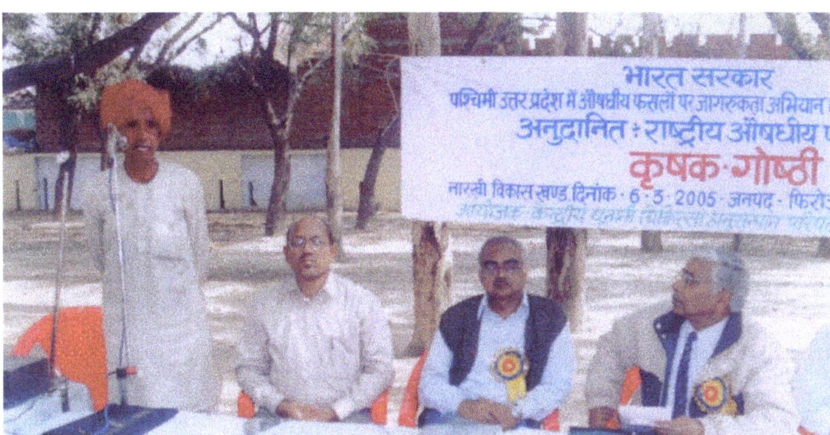

Fig 2: A Farmer Sharing his Experience of Cultivating Medicinal Crops in a Farmers' Meet in Narkhi Development Block at Firozabad on 6th May 2005. Sitting on the Dais are Dr. A.K. Tomar, Marketing Expert, Dr. A.K.S. Chauhan, Agrotechniques expert, Dr. V.K. Singh, Project Director (left to right).

Credits:

The following individuals and organizations contributed to this project:

Financial Assistance:

National Medicinal Plants Board (NMPB), Ministry of AYUSH,

Government of India, New Delhi

Strategic Planning and Implementation:

Dr. R.B.S. Rawat, IFS, CEO, National Medicinal Plants Board

Shri B.S. Sajwan, IFS, CEO, National Medicinal Plants Board

Project Contributors:

- Dr. (Ms.) Shamima Hashmi,Ph.D (Botany), Co-Principal Investigator
  Regional Research Institute of Unani Medicine (CCRUM) – Government of India, Aligarh 202001
- Dr. A.K.S. Chauhan,Ph.D (Botany), Agrotechniques Expert
  D.S. College, Aligarh 202001
- Dr. A.K. Tomar,Ph.D (Economics) Economics Expert
  D.S. College, Aligarh 202001
- Professor Shweta Yadav, Ph.D (Zoology), Vermitechnology Expert
  University of Sagar, M.P. 470002
- Shri R.P.P. Singh, Agriculture Officer
  Government of Rajasthan, Jaipur
- Shri Indra Pal Singh, Accounts and Finance Expert
  Government of U.P. , Lucknow

DEDICATION

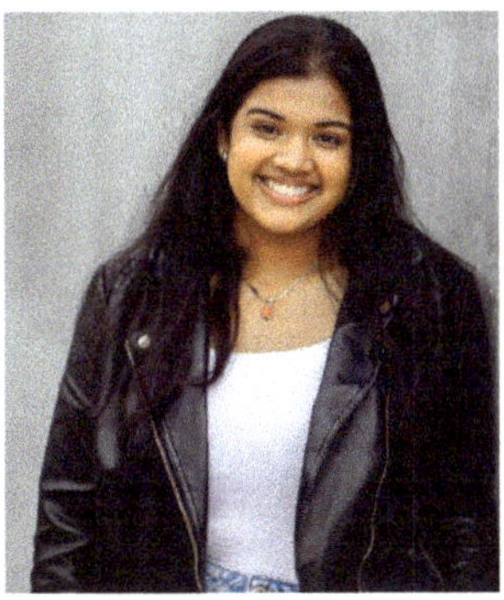

Yashi

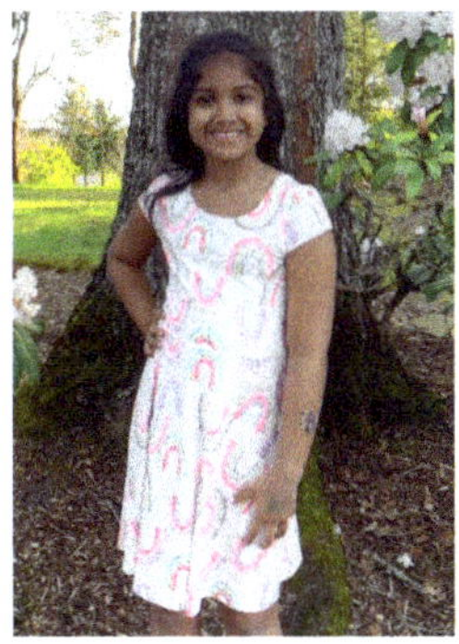

Anika

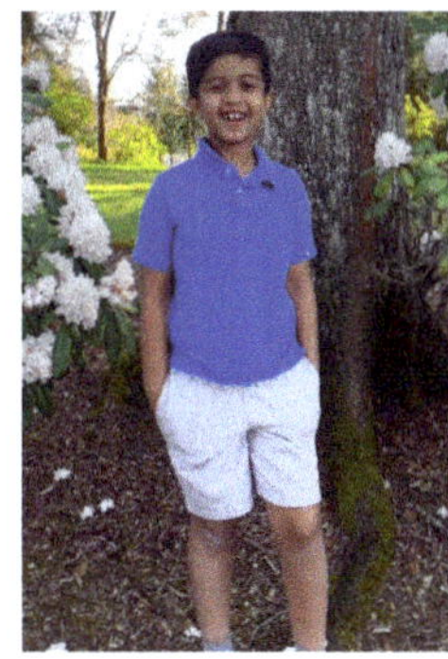

Arush

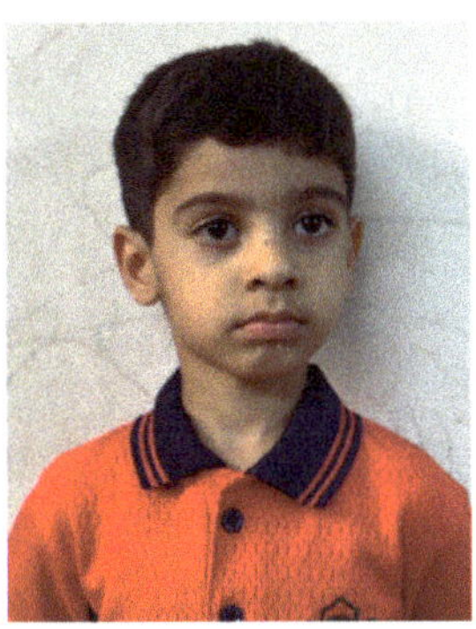

Ashwin

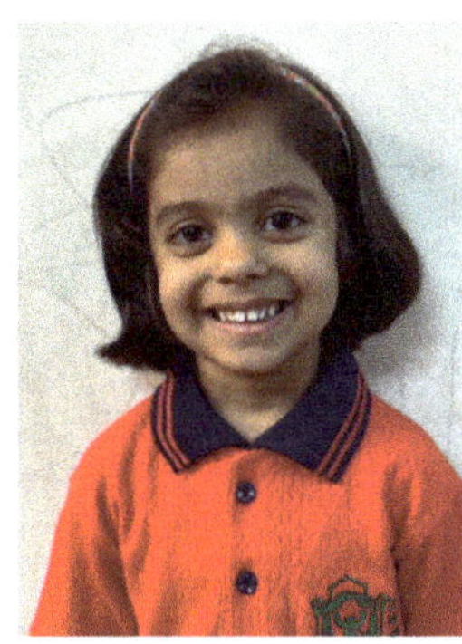

Aaradhya

"To my Dear Grandchildren, Yashi, Arush, Anika, Ashwin, and Aaradhya, with love, blessings, and best wishes – V.K. Singh"

ACKNOWLEDGMENTS

This endeavor would not have been possible without the support of numerous individuals and organizations. I extend my heartfelt gratitude to all, particularly the pioneering farmers of Western UP, who ventured into cultivating medicinal crops alongside traditional ones.

I am grateful for the consistent support and contributions from former officials at the Ministry of AYUSH, Government of India, New Delhi Shri Vijay Singh, IAS, Secretary, Dr. Anis Ahmad Ansari, Adviser, and Dr. M.K. Siddiqui, DG, CCRUM, who provided valuable inputs and wrote prefaces for various publications released during the program period 2002-2006. The author is indebted to the former Chief Executive Officers of the National Medicinal Plants Board, Dr. R.B.S Rawat, IFS, and Mr. B.S. Sajwan, IFS, for their valuable time, guidance, and support in facilitating regular visits to medicinal crop cultivation projects in Western UP villages, encouraging farmers, and lending official sanction to the initiatives.

The medicinal plants data on various aspects presented in this book draws heavily from the research conducted by various organizations including Ministry of AYUSH, Government of India; Centre for Research, Planning, and Action (CERPA); Department of ISM & H and WHO ; National Medicinal Plants Board, New Delhi, and allied sources which have enriched the contents of this book. I sincerely acknowledge all the sources for their valuable contributions.

I extend my sincere thanks to the Regional Research Institute of Unani Medicine (CCRUM), Aligarh, for providing basic facilities to run the project, specifically to Dr. R.S. Verma, Research Officer (Biochemistry), for his expertise in computer typesetting and manuscript uploading, and to Mr. Mohd. Zahid Ansari, Investigator (Statistics), for his meticulous scanning and quality review of the photographs.

Finally, I extend my sincere gratitude to Ms. Yashi Singh, graduated from Northeastern University, Boston, USA with a degree in Behavioral Neuroscience, for her invaluable contributions, expert suggestions, and meticulous formatting that transformed the manuscript into a press-ready document.

EXECUTIVE SUMMARY

The National Medicinal Plants Board (NMPB), Ministry of AYUSH, Government of India, funded the initiative titled *"Medicinal Crops Cultivation in Western Uttar Pradesh, India: Awareness and Training to Farmers."* The project aimed to improve the livelihoods of rural farmers by introducing field-scale cultivation of high-demand medicinal plants suited to the region's agro-climatic conditions.

Conducted from 2002 to 2006, this comprehensive program included multiple integrated activities designed to educate, train, and empower farmers. These included documentation of agrotechnical literature, farmers' meets and workshops, national-level seminars, and the development of model demonstration plots. Additionally, it created a self-sustaining framework involving the distribution of high-quality planting materials, training on vermicompost production, setting up medicinal seed villages, and compiling marketing directory to address commercialization challenges.

By the conclusion of the project, 162 acres of farmland across Western Uttar Pradesh—including Aligarh, Hathras, Etah, and Firozabad—had been brought under medicinal crops cultivation. More than 400 farmers were provided with quality, certified planting materials, and over 3,000 received training in agrotechniques, post-harvest handling, and marketing practices.

A follow-up survey conducted in 2022–2023 confirmed that around 150 farmers in districts like Aligarh, Mathura, Bulandshahar, Agra, and Hapur were actively growing medicinal crops such as Ashwagandha,

Kalmegh, Shatavari, Isabgol, and others, generating good profits on 0.5 to 1 hectare of land.

One of the landmark achievements of this program was the signing of a Memorandum of Understanding (MoU) between the NMPB and ISM pharmaceutical industries on September 24, 2020, ensuring a buyback guarantee for farmers cultivating medicinal crops, to a limited extent. This strategic intervention addressed one of the biggest concerns of farmers—lack of assured buyers and fair pricing.

The program advocated the organized cultivation of 23 priority medicinal species including Milk Thistle, Stevia, Ashwagandha, Isabgol, Mulethi, Kalmegh, Tulsi, and Safed Musli, all recognized for their commercial value and therapeutic potential.

Furthermore, a booklet titled *"Paschimi Uttar Pradesh Mein Aushdhiya Phaslon Ki Kheti—Vikas avum Sambhavana"* was published in Hindi to assist farmers with practical guidance on cultivation practices, economic returns, post-harvest storage, pest management, and the national demand for medicinal raw materials.

Through a structured, multi-dimensional strategy, this initiative demonstrated that medicinal plants cultivation is a viable avenue for enhancing farmer incomes, conserving plant biodiversity, and strengthening India's traditional medicine sector. With continued support from the government and industry stakeholders, this model holds promise for replication across other agro-climatic regions in India.

TABLE OF CONTENTS

PREFACE

Assured and Fair Prices: A Key to Success for Medicinal Crops in India

Traditional medicine continues to play a vital role in addressing emerging health challenges across the world. According to the World Health Organization (WHO), approximately 80% of the global population relies on traditional medicine for primary healthcare. In India, systems such as Ayurveda, Unani, Siddha, and Yoga & Naturopathy—predominantly plant-based—have long formed the backbone of indigenous healing practices.

In recent years, increasing concerns over the side effects of modern pharmaceuticals have accelerated global interest in herbal medicines. Consequently, the demand for herbal raw materials has surged, creating an urgent need for their large-scale cultivation. The sustainability of the AYUSH pharmaceutical industry depends on a consistent and high-quality supply of these medicinal crops.

Driven by this necessity and following exponential growth in the AYUSH sector—from USD 2.85 billion in 2014 to USD 23 billion in 2023—the Hon'ble Prime Minister of India, Shri Narendra Modi, emphasized during a Ministry of AYUSH review meeting on February 27, 2025, the importance of encouraging commercial cultivation of medicinal crops. This initiative aims to uplift the rural economy and improve farmers' livelihoods.

This book is the outcome of a Government of India-funded project under the National Medicinal Plants Board (NMPB), titled *"Medicinal*

Crops Cultivation in Western Uttar Pradesh, India: Awareness and Training to Farmers." The study offers a blueprint for aspiring farmers and agri-entrepreneurs across the country, especially those based in Western Uttar Pradesh, to adopt medicinal crop farming as a profitable and sustainable agricultural venture.

From 2002 to 2006, the project carried out various field-level interventions: establishment of an Information and Facilitation Center in Aligarh, preparation and distribution of literature on agrotechnological methods and marketing in Hindi, organization of farmers' awareness meetings, and a national symposium on advanced agrotechniques and marketing strategies. Key demonstrations included vermicompost use, interactive stakeholder meetings, distribution of high-quality planting materials, pilot studies on local demand, and the setting-up of 35 demonstration plots. Two Medicinal Seed Villages were also established to help farmers become self-reliant in producing their own planting material.

As a direct result of these efforts, 162 acres of land were reclaimed for the first time in Western Uttar Pradesh for the cultivation of medicinal crops. Over 200 farmers were provided organically certified planting materials, and approximately 3,000 farmers were trained on best practices in agrotechniques and marketing strategies.

Medicinal crop farming is not only economically beneficial due to its low cultivation costs and high market value, but it is also ecologically sound. These crops can grow on marginal lands, require minimal irrigation and no chemical fertilizers, and need very little maintenance. Their cultivation helps conserve forest biodiversity by reducing reliance on wild harvesting.

Furthermore, a significant breakthrough was achieved through the signing of Memoranda of Understanding (MoUs) between leading herbal industries and the Government of India, providing farmers with buyback guarantees at fair prices. This development addresses one of the major obstacles faced by farmers: lack of assured marketing mechanisms.

From personal experience, undertaking this initiative was both challenging and fulfilling. Initially, there was widespread skepticism among farmers, as the idea of cultivating medicinal crops was entirely unfamiliar in this region. Considerable effort went into building trust with local farmers, village heads, and key opinion leaders (KOLs). However, as awareness grew, the farming community became increasingly enthusiastic and committed. Their dedication and willingness to follow technical guidance played a crucial role in the program's success.

Despite this progress, much more needs to be done. The government must continue to strengthen the buyback ecosystem and promote long-term partnerships between growers and pharmaceutical manufacturers.

Regretfully, lack of standardized pricing mechanism and Minimum Support Price (MSP) for medicinal crops in India creates uncertainty for farmers and industry stakeholders. To address this, the government needs to establish a fair pricing framework to ensure the sustainability of medicinal crops cultivation.

It is my earnest hope that this book serves as both an informative guide and an inspiration to policymakers, researchers, and farmers alike. Medicinal farming represents a unique opportunity not only to improve rural incomes but also to contribute to sustainable agriculture, biodiversity conservation, and national health resilience.

Dr. V.K. Singh
Project Director & Former Deputy Director (Botany)
CCRUM Headquarters, Ministry of AYUSH, New Delhi
20th June 2025

PROLOGUE

Walking the Rocky Path

Medicinal plants continue to hold immense significance for human health, cultural heritage, and community welfare. Across numerous indigenous and rural communities, these plants are integral to both healthcare and livelihoods. Their cultivation, harvesting, processing, utilization, and trade collectively contribute to the socio-economic upliftment of farming populations.

Globally, it is estimated that nearly 80% of people depend on traditional medicinal systems. The commercial market for herbal and botanical products is projected to exceed USD 72 billion, reflecting a marked increase in demand (Shakya, 2016; Rathore and Mathur, 2018). For small and marginal farmers, cultivating medicinal plants offers a viable diversification strategy. It promises growing trade opportunities, better profit margins, and greater economic stability (Marshall, 2011).

However, several persistent challenges hinder the widespread adoption of medicinal plant cultivation:

(i) Medicinal farming is still perceived as non-remunerative by many farmers due to lack of organized support.
(ii) Absence of assured marketing mechanisms continues to dissuade growers; contract farming agreements remain scarce.
(iii) There is limited farmer knowledge and inadequate training in post-harvest handling of medicinal produce, affecting quality and profitability.

(iv) Adherence to Good Agricultural Practices (GAP) is crucial for sustainable development in the medicinal plant sector, including ecological and preventive cultivation measures.
(v) Most critically, awareness levels about the potential of medicinal crops remain low. Targeted awareness and skill-building programs are urgently needed to bridge this gap.

The purpose of this book is to address these very issues by documenting a structured initiative carried out in Western Uttar Pradesh between 2002 and 2006. It chronicles the real-world experiences, constraints, and successes observed while introducing medicinal farming to a region where it was previously unheard of.

The book aims to offer readers—especially farmers, policymakers, and stakeholders in the AYUSH sector—comprehensive insights into the process, challenges, and potential of cultivating medicinal crops. By learning from this pioneering effort, similar models can be adapted and expanded across other parts of India where agro-climatic conditions are conducive.

It is our conviction that organized, informed, and policy-backed cultivation of medicinal crops will serve as a catalyst for both economic transformation and ecological resilience in India's rural heartland.

GOVERNMENT RECOGNITION AND ENDORSEMENT:

This ambitious project on cultivation and marketing of high-demand medicinal crops in Western UP received consistent support and encouragement from various former officials of the Ministry of AYUSH.

Prefaces to the Publications:

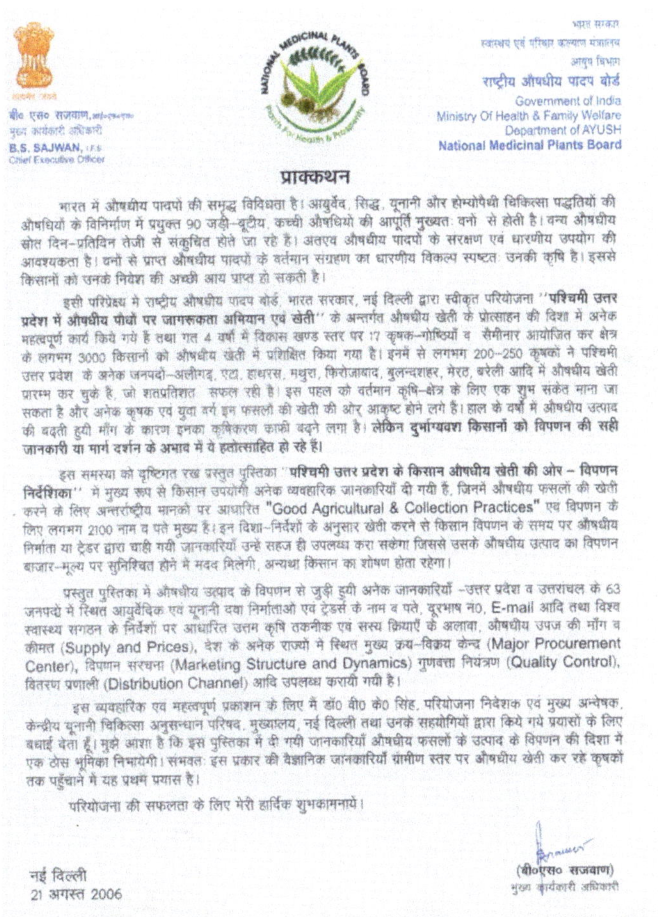

सत्यमेव जयते

बी० एस० सजवाण, आई०एफ०एस०
मुख्य कार्यकारी अधिकारी
B.S. SAJWAN, I.F.S.
Chief Executive Officer

भारत सरकार
स्वास्थ्य एवं परिवार कल्याण मंत्रालय
आयुष विभाग
राष्ट्रीय औषधीय पादप बोर्ड
Government of India
Ministry Of Health & Family Welfare
Department of AYUSH
National Medicinal Plants Board

प्राक्कथन

भारत में औषधीय पादपों की समृद्ध विविधता है। आयुर्वेद, सिद्ध, यूनानी और होम्योपैथी चिकित्सा पद्धतियों की औषधियों के विनिर्माण में प्रयुक्त 90 जड़ी-बूटीय, कच्ची औषधियों की आपूर्ति मुख्यतः वनों से होती है। वन्य औषधीय स्रोत दिन-प्रतिदिन तेजी से संकुचित होते जा रहे हैं। अतएव औषधीय पादपों के संरक्षण एवं धारणीय उपयोग की आवश्यकता है। वनों से प्राप्त औषधीय पादपों के वर्तमान संग्रहण का धारणीय विकल्प स्पष्टतः उनकी कृषि है। इससे किसानों को उनके निवेश की अच्छी आय प्राप्त हो सकती है।

इसी परिप्रेक्ष्य मे राष्ट्रीय औषधीय पादप बोर्ड, भारत सरकार, नई दिल्ली द्वारा स्वीकृत परियोजना ''**पश्चिमी उत्तर प्रदेश में औषधीय पौधों पर जागरूकता अभियान एवं खेती**'' के अन्तर्गत औषधीय खेती के प्रोत्साहन की दिशा में अनेक महत्वपूर्ण कार्य किये गये हैं तथा गत 4 वर्षों में विकास खण्ड स्तर पर 17 कृषक-गोष्ठियाँ व सैमीनार आयोजित कर क्षेत्र के लगभग 3000 किसानों को औषधीय खेती में प्रशिक्षित किया गया है। इनमें से लगभग 200-250 कृषकों ने पश्चिमी उत्तर प्रदेश के अनेक जनपदों-अलीगढ़, एटा, हाथरस, मथुरा, फिरोजाबाद, बुलन्दशहर, मेरठ, बरेली आदि में औषधीय खेती प्रारम्भ कर चुके है, जो शतप्रतिशत सफल रही है। इस पहल को वर्तमान कृषि-क्षेत्र के लिए एक शुभ संकेत माना जा सकता है और अनेक कृषक एवं युवा वर्ग इन फसलों की खेती की ओर आकृष्ट होने लगे हैं। हाल के वर्षों में औषधीय उत्पाद की बढ़ती हुयी माँग के कारण इनका कृषिकरण काफी बढ़ने लगा है। **लेकिन दुर्भाग्यवश किसानों को विपणन की सही जानकारी या मार्ग दर्शन के अभाव में वे हतोत्साहित हो रहे हैं।**

इस समस्या को दृष्टिगत रख प्रस्तुत पुस्तिका ''**पश्चिमी उत्तर प्रदेश के किसान औषधीय खेती की ओर – विपणन निर्देशिका**'' में मुख्य रूप से किसान उपयोगी अनेक व्यवहारिक जानकारियाँ दी गयी हैं, जिनमें औषधीय फसलों की खेती करने के लिए अन्तर्राष्ट्रीय मानकों पर आधारित "Good Agricultural & Collection Practices" एवं विपणन के लिए लगभग 2100 नाम व पते मुख्य हैं। इन दिशा-निर्देशों के अनुसार खेती करने से किसान विपणन के समय पर औषधीय निर्माता या ट्रेडर द्वारा चाही गयी जानकारियाँ उन्हें सहज ही उपलब्ध करा सकेगा जिससे उसके औषधीय उत्पाद का विपणन बाजार-मूल्य पर सुनिश्चित होने में मदद मिलेगी, अन्यथा किसान का शोषण होता रहेगा।

प्रस्तुत पुस्तिका मे औषधीय उत्पाद के विपणन से जुड़ी हुयी अनेक जानकारियाँ -उत्तर प्रदेश व उत्तरांचल के 63 जनपदों में स्थित आयुर्वेदिक एवं यूनानी दवा निर्माताओं एवं ट्रेडर्स के नाम व पते, दूरभाष नं0, E-mail आदि तथा विश्व स्वास्थ्य सगठन के निर्देशों पर आधारित उत्तम कृषि तकनीक एवं सस्य क्रियाएँ के अलावा, औषधीय उपज की माँग व कीमत (Supply and Prices), देश के अनेक राज्यों मे स्थित मुख्य क्रय-विक्रय केन्द (Major Procurement Center), विपणन सरचना (Marketing Structure and Dynamics) गुणवत्ता नियंत्रण (Quality Control), वितरण प्रणाली (Distribution Channel) आदि उपलब्ध करायी गयी है।

इस व्यवहारिक एवं महत्वपूर्ण प्रकाशन के लिए मैं डॉ0 वी0 के0 सिंह, परियोजना निदेशक एवं मुख्य अन्वेषक, केन्द्रीय यूनानी चिकित्सा अनुसन्धान परिषद, मुख्यालय, नई दिल्ली तथा उनके सहयोगियों द्वारा किये गये प्रयासों के लिए बधाई देता हूँ। मुझे आशा है कि इस पुस्तिका में दी गयी जानकारियाँ औषधीय फसलों के उत्पाद के विपणन की दिशा में एक ठोस भूमिका निभायेगी। संभवतः इस प्रकार की वैज्ञानिक जानकारियाँ ग्रामीण स्तर पर औषधीय खेती कर रहे कृषकों तक पहुँचाने में यह प्रथम प्रयास है।

परियोजना की सफलता के लिए मेरी हार्दिक शुभकामनायें।

नई दिल्ली
21 अगस्त 2006

(बी०एस० सजवाण)
मुख्य कार्यकारी अधिकारी

Fig 1:Preface to the Booklet on Marketing Directory of Farmers' Medicinal Produce (2006) by Mr. B.S. Sajwan IFS, former CEO of National Medicinal Plants Board, New Delhi

विजय सिंह
Vijay Singh

सचिव
भारत सरकार
स्वास्थ्य एवं परिवार कल्याण मंत्रालय
आयुर्वेद, योग व प्राकृतिक चिकित्सा,
यूनानी, सिद्ध एवं होम्योपैथी (आयुष) विभाग
रैड क्रॉस भवन, नई दिल्ली - 110001

SECRETARY
GOVERNMENT OF INDIA
MINISTRY OF HEALTH & FAMILY WELFARE
DEPTT. OF AYURVEDA, YOGA & NATUROPATHY,
UNANI, SIDDHA AND HOMOEOPATHY (AYUSH)
RED CROSS BUILDING, NEW DELHI- 110001
Tel. : 011-23715564, Telefax : 011-23327660
E-mail : sec-ismh@nic.in

संदेश

मुझे यह जानकर अत्यंत प्रसन्नता है कि राष्ट्रीय औषधीय पादप बोर्ड, आयुष विभाग, नई दिल्ली, द्वारा प्रायोजित परियोजना के अन्तर्गत **पश्चिमी उत्तर प्रदेश में औषधीय फसलों की खेती (सम्भावना एवं विकास)** पुस्तिका का द्वितीय संशोधित संस्करण प्रकाशित किया जा रहा है। पुस्तिका में मुख्य रूप से पश्चिमी उत्तर प्रदेश की जलवायु के अनुरूप कृषिकरण एवं विपणन हेतु भारतीय चिकित्सा पद्धति में अत्यधिक माँग वाली चिन्हांकित 23 औषधीय प्रजातियों पर किसान उपयोगी अनेक महत्वपूर्ण जानकारियाँ दी गयी हैं।

इस महत्वपूर्ण प्रकाशन के लिए मैं डा0 मौहम्मद खालिद सिद्दकी, निदेशक, केन्द्रीय यूनानी चिकित्सा अनुसंधान परिषद् एवं मुख्य अन्वेषक डॉ0 वी0 के0 सिंह, सहायक निदेशक (वनस्पति), केन्द्रीय यूनानी चिकित्सा अनुसंधान परिषद, मुख्यालय, नई दिल्ली, को बधाई देता हूँ और आशा करता हूँ कि प्रदेश में औषधीय खेती प्रारम्भ करने वाले कृषकों के लिये यह पुस्तिका अत्यंत उपयोगी होगी और औषधीय पादप क्षेत्र के समग्र विकास में महत्वपूर्ण भूमिका निभाएगी।

परियोजना की सफलता के लिये मेरी हार्दिक शुभकामनायें।

28 मार्च, 2006

(विजय सिंह)

Fig 2: Appreciation Message to the Booklet on Agrotechniqures and Marketing of High Demand Medicinal Crops in Western UP (2006) by Shri Vijay Singh, IAS, Former Secretary to the Government of India, New Delhi

बी० एस० सजवाण, आई०एफ०एस०
मुख्य कार्यकारी अधिकारी
B.S. SAJWAN, I.F.S.
Chief Executive Officer

भारत सरकार
स्वास्थ्य एवं परिवार कल्याण मंत्रालय
आयुष विभाग
राष्ट्रीय औषधीय पादप बोर्ड
Government of India
Ministry Of Health & Family Welfare
Department of AYUSH
National Medicinal Plants Board

प्राक्कथन

आदिकाल से ही भारत की ग्रामीण जनता एवं जनजातियाँ अपने रोगों और स्वास्थ्य हेतु दिन–प्रतिदिन की जरूरतों के लिये आसपास के पादपों/जंगलों पर निर्भर रहती आयी है। आयुर्वेद, सिद्ध, यूनानी और होम्योपैथी चिकित्सा पद्धतियों की औषधियों के विनिर्माण में प्रयुक्त 90 प्रतिशत जड़ी–बूटीय कच्ची औषधियों की आपूर्ति मुख्यतः वनों से होती है। आज औषधीय पादप न केवल स्वास्थ्य परिचर्या के स्रोत के रूप में वरन् आय के स्रोत के रूप में भी स्वीकार किये जा रहे हैं।

वन्य स्रोत दिन प्रतिदिन तेजी से संकुचित होते जा रहे हैं। अतएव औषधीय पादपों के संरक्षण एवं धारणीय उपयोग की आवश्यकता है। वनों से प्राप्त औषधीय पादपों के वर्तमान संग्रहण का धारणीय विकल्प स्पष्टतः उनकी कृषि है, इससे किसानों को उनके निवेश की अच्छी आय प्राप्त हो सकती है। भारत के औषधीय पादपों से सम्बन्धित व्यापार का मूल्य 2004-2005 वित्तीय वर्ष मे लगभग 180 मिलियन अमरेकी डालर (निर्यात – आयात बैंक) है और यह दिन प्रतिदिन बढ़ रहा है। वर्तमान में जड़ी बूटीय उत्पादों का अन्तर्राष्ट्रीय बाजार 62 बिलियन अमेरीकी डालर तक होने का अनुमान है तथा सन् 2050 तक 5 ट्रिलियन डालर होने की पूर्ण संभावना है (विश्व बैंक रिपोर्ट, 1996)।

वस्तुतः कृषिकरण की दृष्टि से वर्तमान समय को जड़ी–बूटियों का स्वर्णिम युग माना जाये तो कोई अतिश्योक्ति नही होगी क्योंकि एक तरफ जहाँ इनकी खेती हेतु विधिवत प्रशिक्षण की व्यवस्था होने लगी है वहीं इनकी खेती के लिये बैंकों द्वारा उदारतापूर्वक ऋण भी प्रदान किया जाने लगा है। इस दिशा मे राष्ट्रीय औषधीय पादप बोर्ड, नई दिल्ली द्वारा किसानों को औषधीय खेती के लिये 9 लाख रूपये तक की वित्तीय सहायता का प्रावधान है। प्रदेश के कृषकों के लिये यह हर्ष की बात है कि भारतीय चिकित्सा पद्धतियों में बहुतायत से उपयोग होने वाली जिन 20 औषधीय प्रजातियों की देश में आन्तरिक माँग शीर्ष स्तर पर है उनमे से 18 का कृषिकरण पश्चिमी उत्तर प्रदेश की जलवायु में आसानी से किया जा सकता है। इन फसलों की खेती कर क्षेत्र के किसान शीघ्र ही आर्थिक रूप से लाभान्वित हो सकते हैं। हाल में किये गये एक अध्ययन (2003) के अनुसार देश की वर्ष 2004–05 की आन्तरिक माँग के अनुसार इनमें प्रमुख प्रजातियाँ हैं : **आँवला** (34568.8 टन); **अश्वगन्धा** (9127.2 टन); **अशोक** (10724.2 टन); **सनाय** (9828.2 टन); **ब्रह्मी** (2650.1 टन); **पुर्ननवा** (3373.2 टन); **मकोय** (2192.2 टन); **कालमेघ** (2197.3 टन), **शतावर** (16615 टन); **हरण** (6778 टन); **बेल** (7084.5 टन), **अडूसा** (7065.4 टन); **तुलसी** (5014.0 टन);, **नीम** (5241.6 टन); **धाय** (3760.7 टन); **गिलोय** (2932.6 टन) (2004–05 की अनुमानित मांग)। केवल आवश्यकता है इन औषधीय फसलों के उत्पाद के संचालित विपणन की। इस दिशा में परियोजना द्वारा आवश्यक प्रयास किये जा रहे है और आशा है परिणाम उत्साहजनक होंगे।

परियोजना के अन्तर्गत वर्ष 2002-2006 में पश्चिमी उत्तर प्रदेश मे औषधीय पादपों के विकास एवं कृषिकरण से सम्बन्धित अनेक महत्वपूर्ण कार्य किये गये है जिनमे प्रमुख हैं– भारतीय चिकित्सा पद्धति में बहुतायत से प्रयुक्त महत्वपूर्ण औषधीय प्रजातियों की खेती से सम्बन्धित साहित्य तैयार करना; विकास एवं जिला स्तर पर औषधीय पादपों पर जागरूकता अभियान के अन्तर्गत क्षेत्र मे अनेक कृषक गोष्ठियाँ आयोजित कर कृषकों को आवश्यक जानकारी उपलब्ध कराना; उन्नतशील कृषकों का चयन कर औषधीय खेती पर विशेष प्रशिक्षण दिलवाना; औषधीय प्रजातियों (**सनाय, कालमेघ, अश्वगन्धा, गुलेनार, जैट्रोफा, कौंच, मुश्कदाना, आँवला, बेल**) पर कृषकों के स्वयं के खेतों पर **''प्रदर्शन प्लाट''** आयोजित करना; और औषधीय पादपों की वृहद स्तर पर खेती हेतु क्षेत्र के कृषकों को उत्तम किस्म के बीज दिलवाना, बहुस्तरीय औषधि खेती, औषधीय फसलों की बीमारियों का उपचार, औषधीय उपज के विपणन मे मार्गदर्शन एवं उत्तर प्रदेश के अलीगढ़ जनपद में प्रथम ''औषधीय बीज गाँव'' की स्थापना आदि शामिल है। **हर्ष की बात है कि प्रारम्भ से ही निरंतर उत्कृष्ट कार्य के लिये इस परियोजना को औषधीय पादप बोर्ड, नई दिल्ली द्वारा वर्ष 2003-04 व 2004-05 के लिये श्रेष्ठ स्तर पर आँका गया है।**

इसी परिप्रेक्ष्य में प्रस्तुत पुस्तिका **''पश्चिमी उत्तर प्रदेश में औषधीय फसलों की खेती - सम्भावना एंव विकास''** के संशोधित द्वितीय संस्करण में कृषि उपयोगी अनेक विषयों पर महत्वपूर्ण एवं व्यवहारिक जानकारी दी गयी है जो एक प्रशंसनीय प्रयास है। मुझे आशा है कि ये सभी जानकारियाँ क्षेत्र के कृषकों को औषधीय फसलों की खेती प्रारम्भ करने में लाभकारी होंगी और पश्चिमी उत्तर प्रदेश में औषधीय पादप क्षेत्र को विकसित करने में सभी पणधारियों (उत्पादकों, संग्रहणकर्ताओं, व्यापारियों, आयुर्वेदिक एवं यूनानी औषधि निर्माताओं) के लिये उपयोगी होगी।

मुझे इस पुस्तिका का प्राक्कथन लिखने में अत्यधिक खुशी एवं गर्व महसूस हो रहा है और इस प्रयास के लिये मैं डा० वी०के० सिंह, परियोजना निदेशक एवं डा० (श्रीमती) शमीमा हाशमी, सह मुख्य अन्वेषक एवं समस्त कार्यदल को बधाई देता हूँ और उत्सुकतापूर्वक आशा करता हूँ कि इस पुस्तिका में दी गयी जानकारी पश्चिमी उत्तर प्रदेश के कृषकों के लिये अत्यन्त लाभकारी होगी तथा औषधीय फसलों के विकास एवं कृषिकरण को एक नई दिशा मिलेगी।

मैं परियोजना की सफलता की कामना करता हूँ।

9 मार्च, 2006

(बी०एस० सजवाण)
मुख्य कार्यकारी अधिकारी

Fig 3:Preface to the Booklet on Agrotechniques of High Demand Medicinal Crops, in Western Uttar Pradesh (2006) by Mr. B.S. Sajwan IFS, former CEO, National Medicinal Plants Board, New Delhi

सत्यमेव जयते

Prof. Anis A. Ansari
ADVISOR (UNANI)
Tel. : 3325799

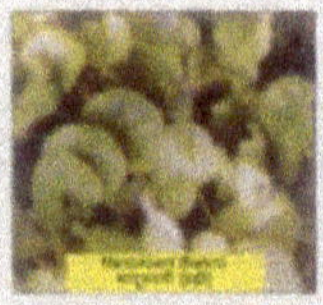

MEDICINAL PLANTS
FOR HEALTHY
LIVING

भारत सरकार
स्वास्थ्य एवं परिवार कल्याण मंत्रालय
भारतीय चिकित्सा पद्धति एवं होमियोपैथिक विभाग
रेडक्रोस भवन, नई दिल्ली-११०००१

GOVERNMENT OF INDIA
MINISTRY OF HEALTH & FAMILY WELFARE
DEPTT. OF ISM & HOMOEOPATHY
REDCROSS BUILDING, NEW DELHI-110001

प्राक्कथन

आदिकाल से ही भारत की ग्रामीण जनता एवं जनजातियाँ अपने रोगों और स्वास्थ्य हेतु दिन–प्रतिदिन की जरूरतों के लिये आसपास के पादपों/जंगलों पर निर्भर रहती आयी है। आयुर्वेद, सिद्ध, यूनानी और होम्योपैथी चिकित्सा पद्धतियों की औषधियों के विनिर्माण में प्रयुक्त ९० प्रतिशत जड़ी–बूटीय कच्ची औषधियों की आपूर्ति मुख्यतः वनों से होती है। आज औषधीय पादप न केवल स्वास्थ्य परिचर्या के स्रोत के रूप में वरन् आय के स्रोत के रूप मे भी स्वीकार किये जा रहे हैं।

वन्य स्रोत दिन प्रतिदिन तेजी से संकुचित होते जा रहे हैं। अतएव औषधीय पादपों के संरक्षण एवं धारणीय उपयोग की आवश्यकता है। वनों से प्राप्त औषधीय पादपों के वर्तमान संग्रहण का धारणीय विकल्प स्पष्टतः उनकी कृषि है, इससे किसानों को उनके निवेश की अच्छी आय प्राप्त हो सकती है। भारत के औषधीय पादपों से सम्बन्धित व्यापार का मूल्य ५.५ बिलियन अमेरिकी डालर (निर्यात – आयात बैंक प्रतिवेदन १९९७) है और यह दिन प्रतिदिन बढ़ रहा है। वर्तमान में जड़ी बूटीय उत्पादों का अन्तर्राष्ट्रीय बाजार ६२ बिलियन अमेरीकी डालर तक होने का अनुमान है।

देश विदेश में औषधीय पादपों की बढ़ती माँग को देखते हुये इनकी खेती के प्रति किसानों में रूझान तो हुआ है परन्तु जड़ी–बूटियों की खेती कब और कैसे करें, कैसी जलवायु और जमीन पर किसकी खेती लाभप्रद होगी, इस सबकी जानकारी अभी तक पश्चिमी उत्तर प्रदेश के किसानों को न के बराबर है। इसी उद्देश्य से राष्ट्रीय औषधीय पादप बोर्ड, भारत सरकार, नई दिल्ली ने पश्चिमी उत्तर प्रदेश में औषधीय पादपों के कृषिकरण एवं विकास के लिये एक परियोजना स्वीकृत की है जिसका मुख्यालय केन्द्रीय यूनानी चिकित्सा अनुसंधान परिषद, नई दिल्ली है तथा परियोजना का कार्यबिन्दु क्षेत्रीय यूनानी चिकित्सा अनुसंधान संस्थान, अलीगढ़ है।

परियोजना के अन्तर्गत वर्ष २००२–२००३ में पश्चिमी उत्तर प्रदेश में औषधीय पादपों के विकास एवं कृषिकरण से सम्बन्धित अनेक महत्वपूर्ण कार्य किये गये हैं जिनमें प्रमुख हैं– भारतीय चिकित्सा पद्धति में बहुतायत से प्रयुक्त मुख्य औषधीय प्रजातियों की खेती से सम्बन्धित साहित्य तैयार करना; विकास एवं मण्डल स्तर पर औषधीय पादपों पर जागरूकता अभियान के अन्तर्गत क्षेत्र में कृषक गोष्ठियाँ आयोजित कर कृषकों को आवश्यक जानकारी उपलब्ध कराना; उन्नतशील कृषकों का चयन कर औषधीय खेती पर विशेष प्रशिक्षण दिलवाना; औषधीय प्रजातियों (सनाय, कालमेघ, अश्वगन्धा, गुलेनार, जैट्रोफा, कौंच, मुश्कदाना) पर कृषकों के स्वयं के खेतों पर **"प्रदर्शन प्लाट"** आयोजित करवाना, और औषधीय पादपों की वृहद स्तर पर खेती हेतु क्षेत्र के कृषकों को उत्तम किस्म के बीज दिलवाना आदि शामिल है।

इसी परिप्रेक्ष्य में प्रस्तुत पुस्तिका **"औषधीय फसलों की पश्चिमी उत्तर प्रदेश में खेती - सम्भावना और विकास"** में कृषि उपयोगी अनेक विषयों पर महत्वपूर्ण एवं व्यवहारिक जानकारी दी गयी है जो एक प्रशंसनीय प्रयास है। मुझे आशा है कि ये सभी जानकारियाँ क्षेत्र के कृषकों को औषधीय फसलों की खेती प्रारम्भ करने में लाभकारी होंगी और पश्चिमी उत्तर प्रदेश में औषधीय पादप क्षेत्र को विकसित करने में सभी पणधारियों (उत्पादकों, संग्रहणकर्ताओं, व्यापारियों, आयुर्वेदिक एवं यूनानी औषधि निर्माताओं) के लिये उपयोगी होगी।

मुझे इस पुस्तिका का प्राक्कथन लिखने में अत्यधिक खुशी एवं गर्व महसूस हो रहा है और इस प्रयास के लिये मैं डा० वी०के० सिंह, परियोजना निदेशक एवं डा० (श्रीमती) शमीमा हाशमी, सह मुख्य अन्वेषक, को बधाई देता हूँ और उत्सुकतापूर्वक आशा करता हूँ कि इस पुस्तिका में दी गयी जानकारी पश्चिमी उत्तर प्रदेश के कृषकों के लिये अत्यन्त लाभकारी होगी तथा औषधीय फसलों के विकास एवं कृषिकरण को एक नई दिशा मिलेगी। मैं परियोजना की सफलता की कामना करता हूँ।

29.10.2003

अनीस अ. अंसारी
(प्रो० (डॉ०) अनीस अहमद अंसारी)
सलाहकार (यूनानी मैडिसिन) एवं
प्रभारी निदेशक, केन्द्रीय यूनानी चिकित्सा अनुसंधान परिषद,
(भारतीय चिकित्सा पद्धति एवं होम्योपैथी विभाग)
स्वास्थ्य एवं परिवार कल्याण मंत्रालय
भारत सरकार, नई दिल्ली।

Fig 4:Preface to the Booklet on Agrotechniques of High demand Medicinal Crops in Western U.P. (2003)by Dr. A.A. Ansari, former Advisor, Ministry of AYUSH, Government of India, New Delhi

केन्द्रीय यूनानी चिकित्सा अनुसंधान परिषद CCRUM مرکزی کونسل برائے تحقیقات طب یونانی

CENTRAL COUNCIL FOR RESEARCH IN UNANI MEDICINE

An Autonomous Organisation of Ministry of Health and Family Welfare, Government of India
Department of Ayurveda, Yoga & Naturopathy, Unani, Siddha and Homeopathy

Dr. Mohammed Khalid Siddiqui
Director

प्रस्तावना

समग्र स्वास्थ्य हेतु जड़ी–बूटियों की अपरिहार्य आवश्यकता विश्व भर में अनुभव की जा रही है। भारत की औषधीय जैविक विविधता ने सम्पूर्ण विश्व को आकर्षित किया है। यूनानी, आयुर्वेद, सिद्ध, होम्योपैथी तथा एलोपैथी में जड़ी–बूटियों से निर्मित दवाएं जहाँ हानि रहित है वहीं आर्थिक दृष्टि से निर्यात में अत्यन्त लाभकारी हो सकती है। वर्तमान समय में राष्ट्रीय एवं अर्न्तराष्ट्रीय स्तर पर हर्बल उत्पादों एवं जड़ी–बूटियों की मांग में उत्तरोत्तर वृद्धि हो रही है जिसकी पूर्ति के लिए प्राकृतिक जंगलों में उपलब्ध जड़ी–बूटियाँ न केवल अपर्याप्त साबित हो रही हैं बल्कि उनका अत्यधिक अविवेकपूर्ण दोहन होने के कारण कई बहुमूल्य औषधीय पौधों की प्रजातियाँ विलुप्त होने के कगार पर खड़ी हैं। इस समस्या का केवल एक ही विकल्प है कि औषधीय पौधों की व्यवसायिक खेती की जाय। इस दिशा में भारत सरकार ने राष्ट्रीय स्तर पर औषधीय पादप बोर्ड का गठन कर एक अच्छी पहल की है।

इस परिप्रेक्ष्य में केन्द्रीय यूनानी चिकित्सा अनुसंधान परिषद, नई दिल्ली द्वारा संचालित परियोजना ''**पश्चिमी उत्तर प्रदेश में औषधीय पौधों पर जागरूकता अभियान एवं खेती**'' के अन्तर्गत यूनानी एवं आयुर्वेदिक चिकित्सा पद्धति में बृह्द स्तर पर प्रयुक्त विभिन्न औषधीय पौधों की खेती पश्चिमी उत्तर प्रदेश के अनेक जनपदों के किसानों द्वारा वर्ष 2003-06 में की गयी है जिसके उत्साहजनक परिणाम प्राप्त हुये। अभी तक किसानों को उनके औषधीय उत्पाद की बिक्री की सही जानकारी न होने से उन्हें अनेक कठिनाइयों का सामना करना पड़ता है। औषधीय उत्पाद की बिक्री सुनिश्चित करने के लिए आवश्यक है कि औषधीय फसलों की खेती अर्न्तराष्ट्रीय मानकों के आधार पर हो।

जड़ी–बूटियों की बिपणन की समस्या को सामने रखते हुए प्रस्तुत पुस्तिका ''**पश्चिमी उत्तर प्रदेश के किसान औषधीय फसलों की खेती की ओर – विपणन निर्देशिका**'' में औषधीय उत्पाद की राष्ट्रीय एवं अन्तराष्ट्रीय बाजार (विशेषकर उत्तर प्रदेश एवं उत्तरांचल) में बिक्री करने हेतु अनेक जानकारियाँ दी गयी हैं जिन्हें किसानों को खेती प्रारम्भ करने से पूर्व ही पालन करना होगा। इनमें ''**विश्व स्वास्थ्य संगठन**'' द्वारा निर्धारित माप दण्डों के आधार पर सरल हिन्दी में दी गयी ''**अच्छी औषधीय खेती कि सस्य क्रियायें**'' (Good Agricultural and Collection Practices) के दिशा निर्देशों का विशेष महत्व है।

इसके अलावा वर्मीकम्पोस्ट का महत्व व बनाने की विधि, औषधीय उत्पाद की मांग व कीमत, वितरण प्रणाली, राज्यों के मुख्य क्रय–विक्रय केन्द, विपणन संरचना आदि पर सूचनायें संकलित कर सुनियोजित रूप में सरल हिन्दी भाषा में दी गयी है। इनके अलावा औषधीय उत्पाद के विपणन हेतु उत्तर प्रदेश व उत्तरांचल के 63 जनपदों मे स्थित प्रमुख 2100 यूनानी एवं आयुर्वेदिक दवा निर्माताओं, ट्रेडर्स, निर्यातक आदि के नाम, पते, दूरभाष नम्बर व ई–मेल (जहाँ सम्भव है) दिये गये हैं।

इस सम्बन्ध में हम उन सभी संस्थाओं एवं लेखकों के प्रति आभार व्यक्त करते हैं, जिनकी कृतियों से इस कार्य के लिए सामग्री ली गयी। हम राष्ट्रीय औषधीय पादप बोर्ड, नई दिल्ली के परियोजना की वित्तीय सहायता हेतु आभारी हैं।

प्रस्तुत पुस्तिका के प्रकाशन हेतु डा0 वी0 के0 सिंह, मुख्य अन्वेषक एवं सहायक निदेशक (बनस्पति), केन्द्रीय यूनानी चिकित्सा अनुसंधान परिषद, मुख्यालय, नई दिल्ली बधाई के पात्र हैं, जिन्होंने इस पुस्तिका के संकलन मे योगदान दिया। आशा है कि पुस्तिका में उपलब्ध नवीन जानकारियाँ औषधीय फसलों के उत्पाद के विपणन में अत्यन्त लाभकारी होगी।

नई दिल्ली
10 अगस्त, 2006

(डॉ० मोहम्मद खालिद सिद्दीकी)
निदेशक

Fig 5: Preface to the Booklet on Marketing Directory of Farmers' Medicinal Produce (2006) by Dr. M.K. Siddiqui, Director General, CCRUM, Ministry of AYUSH, Government of India, New Delhi

FARMERS' LEAD THE WAY:

Facilitating Officials and Experts on the Successful Completion of Medicinal Crops Cultivation in Western Uttar Pradesh, India, during a Farewell Farmers' Meet at Gabhana in February, 2007

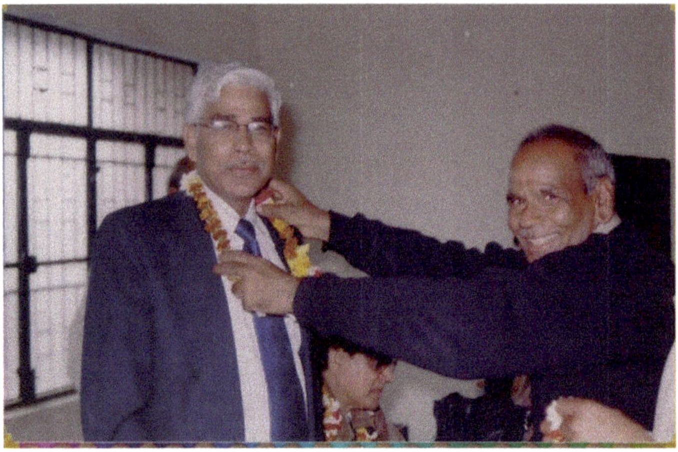

Fig 1: Dr V.K. Singh, Project Director is being Presented with a Garland by a Dedicated Farmer, Mr. Dhyan Pal Singh, Panihavar Village, District Aligarh

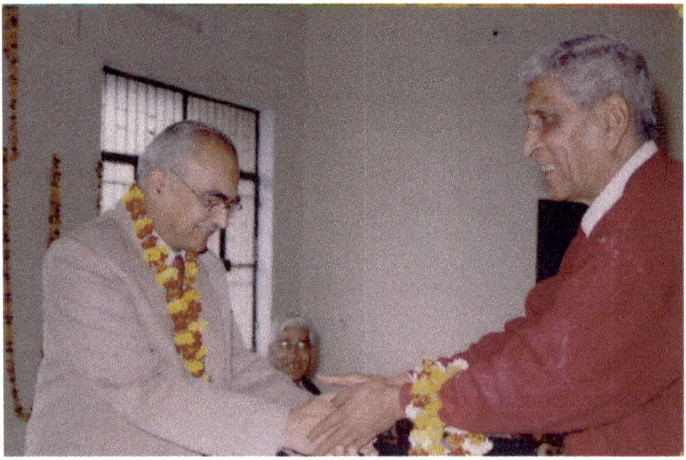

Fig 2: Dr.A.K.S. Chauhan, Expert on Agrotechniques of Medicinal Crops being Presented with a Garland by Mr. R.P.P. Singh, Agriculture Expert

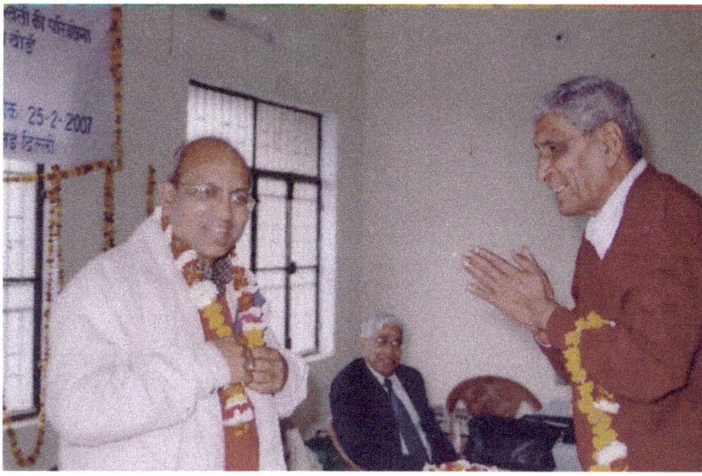

Fig 3: Dr. A.K. Tomar, Expert on Economics of Cultivation of Medicinal Crops being Presented with a Garland by Mr. R.P.P. Singh, Agriculture Expert

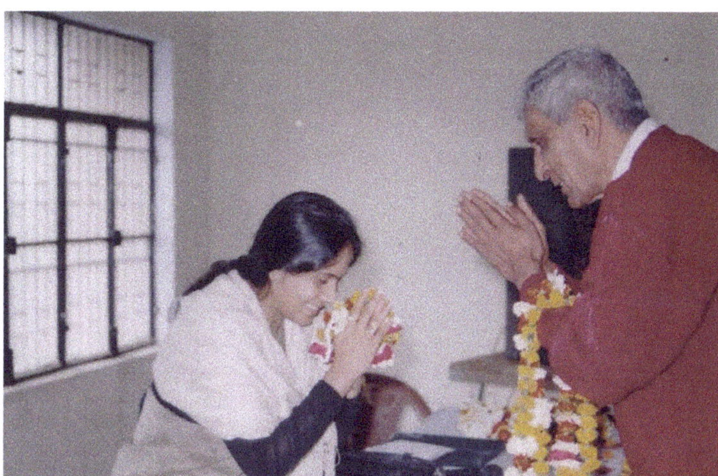

Fig 4: Professor Shweta Yadav, Expert on Vermi technology being Presented with a Garland by Mr. R.P.P. Singh, Agriculture Expert

CHAPTER I

INTRODUCTION

Medicinal plants form the cornerstone of traditional health systems and serve as a major resource for the pharmaceutical industry. These plants provide raw materials for a wide range of therapeutic formulations, from simple home remedies to standardized extracts and active pharmaceutical ingredients. Their importance is steadily rising, especially in the face of growing demand for natural, safe, and affordable healthcare solutions.

There is a global trend towards the resurgence of plant-based medicine, not only as an alternative to synthetic drugs but also as an essential healthcare choice, particularly for economically disadvantaged populations. In this context, herbal medicine is being embraced not just culturally but economically as well, creating significant opportunities for cultivation, processing, and trade.

The increased global demand for herbal medicines has led to a surge in the production of AYUSH products in India. However, this has come at a cost: overexploitation of wild plant species has become a serious issue. Unsustainable harvesting practices have diminished natural populations and biodiversity, leading to concerns over quality, safety, and continuity of raw material supply. Moreover, manufacturers have resorted to using adulterated or substandard materials to meet production demands, compromising the quality of medicines.

The only sustainable alternative is to cultivate medicinal plants on a field scale. This would ensure a steady supply of high-quality raw materials, allow for quality control, and conserve valuable medicinal species in their natural habitats. Recognizing this urgent need, the Government of India launched multiple initiatives to support medicinal plant cultivation, particularly under the AYUSH mission.

1.1 Government's Push to Enhance Farmer Incomes

India's agricultural sector is dominated by small and marginal farmers, with 89.4% owning less than two hectares of land. Average monthly incomes are low, ranging from Rs. 5,298 to Rs. 10,695 nationally, and around Rs. 8,061 in Uttar Pradesh. Persistent debt, crop failures, and low returns have made traditional farming unsustainable for many. In 2016, the Government of India set a goal to double farmers income by 2022. One of the key strategies recommended was agricultural diversification through high-value, market-linked crops.

1.2 Medicinal Crops as an Economic Alternative

Given the high market value and low input costs of medicinal crops, they represent a promising alternative to conventional farming. Their cultivation aligns with the increased demand for standardized herbal products from pharmaceutical industries, both domestically and internationally. This book provides a comprehensive roadmap for farmers wishing to transition to medicinal crops, offering practical guidance on selection, cultivation, processing, and marketing.

1.3 Current Status in Western Uttar Pradesh

A rapid assessment conducted in 2023 found that, even after 18 years since the original project's conclusion, medicinal crop cultivation has gained substantial traction. As of 2022–23, approximately 150 farmers in Aligarh, Mathura, Bulandshahar, and Hapur are cultivating species like Ashwagandha, Kalmegh, Shatavari, Mushkdana, Isabgol, Jatropha, and others on small plots of 0.5–1 hectare.

(A list of 53 farmers cultivating medicinal crops is given in Appendix ii.)

1.4 Step-by-Step Implementation Framework:

The program, implemented from 2002 to 2006, followed a structured model:

- Development of Hindi-language pamphlets detailing agrotechnical practices for 23 prioritized medicinal crops.
- Organization of farmers' awareness meets across rural blocks.
- National seminar introducing advanced techniques and marketing strategies.
- Establishment of 35 village-based demonstration plots.
- Engagement with traders, manufacturers, and ISM stakeholders to ensure market linkages.
- Distribution of high-quality planting material to farmers.
- Specialized training at institutions like the Rajasthan Agro-Forestry Corporation.
- Estimation studies of local demand for medicinal raw materials.
- Initiation of "Field Days" and farmers' interactive events.
- Setup of vermicomposting units for organic input production.
- Publication of handbooks and market directories.
- Establishment of medicinal seed villages to enhance self-reliance.
- Regular oversight and publicity to encourage adoption and visibility.

The results have validated medicinal crops as a sustainable and profitable agricultural pathway. Their inclusion in mainstream farming can boost rural incomes, ensure supply for the AYUSH sector, and promote environmental conservation.

Background and Justification

The strategic promotion of medicinal crop cultivation is rooted in a multifaceted rationale that spans economic, ecological, cultural, and healthcare dimensions. In India, traditional medical systems such as Ayurveda, Unani, Siddha, and Naturopathy—collectively known as AYUSH—rely heavily on plant-based raw materials. Over 90% of AYUSH formulations are derived from medicinal plants, yet most of these resources continue to be harvested from the wild. This practice is unsustainable and endangers both plant biodiversity and quality control.

Recognizing this issue, the Government of India has emphasized the need to transition from wild harvesting to organized cultivation. Through various national missions, including the National AYUSH Mission (NAM) and schemes under the National Medicinal Plants Board (NMPB), concerted efforts are being made to boost the cultivation, processing, and marketing of medicinal crops.

1.5 Growing Global Demand and Trade Potential

Globally, there is a surge in the demand for herbal medicines, nutraceuticals, and wellness products. India's share in the global herbal trade is estimated at around 2.5%, but this figure is poised to grow. Export demand for raw herbs and value-added formulations is rising, especially from countries in Europe, North America, and Southeast Asia.

The Indian herbal industry is valued at over USD 23 billion (as of 2023), with projections suggesting continued growth. However, this growth will only be sustainable if the supply chain—from cultivation to processing—is strengthened through policy support, infrastructure, and farmer participation.

1.6 India's Agro-Climatic Advantage

India possesses vast agro-climatic diversity that supports the cultivation of a wide range of medicinal plant species. From tropical to temperate zones, more than 7,500 plant species are known for their medicinal value. This diversity offers India a comparative advantage in becoming a global leader in the medicinal plant sector.

In states like Uttar Pradesh, where fertile soil, moderate rainfall, and a large agricultural workforce converge, there exists significant untapped potential for medicinal crop farming. Western Uttar Pradesh, in particular, has emerged as a promising region for pilot-scale interventions.

1.7 Unutilized and Marginal Lands

Much of the cultivable land in rural India remains either underutilized or used inefficiently. In Western Uttar Pradesh, many farmers continue to face diminishing returns from traditional crops due to degraded soil, water scarcity, and fluctuating market prices. Medicinal crops, which are hardy, require minimal inputs, and fetch premium prices, can be a game-changer for such regions.

The cultivation of medicinal plants on marginal lands also helps alleviate pressure on forest resources, thus contributing to biodiversity conservation and ecological balance.

1.8 Socioeconomic Impact and Rural Empowerment

Medicinal plant cultivation has the potential to create rural employment opportunities across multiple segments: farming, nursery management, processing, quality control, and marketing. This sector is especially promising for women, smallholder farmers, and landless laborers.

In Western Uttar Pradesh, training programs have already begun to empower rural youth and women's self-help groups. Skill development in medicinal farming is leading to alternative income streams and long-term livelihood security.

1.9 Addressing Farmer Vulnerabilities

Traditional farming is increasingly unviable for small-scale farmers due to rising input costs and erratic climatic patterns. Medicinal crops offer a lower-risk model. Their high market value, coupled with government support and emerging buyback arrangements, presents a viable alternative. Additionally, many medicinal crops are less susceptible to pests and require fewer pesticides, aligning well with organic and sustainable agriculture principles.

1.10 Alignment with National Missions

The cultivation of medicinal plants aligns with several national priorities:

- Doubling Farmers' Income: Promoting high-value crops that are market-linked and environmentally sustainable.
- Make in India: Strengthening indigenous production of raw materials for AYUSH and herbal pharmaceutical industries.
- Atmanirbhar Bharat (Self-Reliant India): Reducing dependency on imported medicinal raw materials.
- Sustainable Development Goals (SDGs): Contributing to poverty alleviation, responsible consumption, and environmental conservation.

Project Design and Implementation Strategy

The project titled *"Medicinal Crops Cultivation in Western Uttar Pradesh: Awareness and Training to Farmers"* was conceptualized as a comprehensive initiative to empower farmers with the knowledge, resources, and institutional support required to cultivate medicinal crops profitably and sustainably. The strategic design encompassed awareness generation, training, demonstration, and facilitation of market linkages.

1.11 Objectives of the Project

The key objectives of the project were:

- To promote awareness among rural farmers about the economic, ecological, and medicinal importance of selected high-value medicinal crops.
- To build farmers' capacity through technical training in cultivation practices, organic farming inputs, and post-harvest management.
- To establish demonstration plots and seed villages to support hands-on learning and promote self-sufficiency in planting material.
- To facilitate interaction between farmers, industry stakeholders, and buyers to ensure reliable marketing channels and fair pricing.

- To document and disseminate field-level agrotechnical practices and marketing insights in a farmer-friendly format.

1.12 Methodology and Approach

The implementation strategy followed a structured, multi-pronged approach:

i. Baseline Assessment and Need Identification:
   The first step involved a rapid assessment to identify suitable districts and farming communities with the potential for medicinal crop adoption. Criteria included land availability, existing agricultural practices, farmer readiness, and regional agro-climatic compatibility.

ii. Awareness Generation:
   Awareness meetings were organized across various blocks in Western Uttar Pradesh. These interactive events focused on:
   - Benefits of medicinal farming compared to conventional crops
   - Ecological sustainability and economic profitability
   - Government support schemes and buyback policies

iii. Training and Capacity Building:
   Training sessions were conducted in partnership with institutions such as the Rajasthan Agro-Forestry Corporation. These sessions covered:
   - Nursery raising techniques
   - Vermicomposting and organic input preparation
   - Good Agricultural Practices (GAP)
   - Pest and disease management in medicinal crops
   - Post-harvest handling, drying, and storage

iv. Demonstration Plots and Field Days:
   Thirty-five demonstration plots were established in selected villages. These served as live field labs where farmers could observe and adopt recommended practices. "Field Days" were also organized, allowing farmers from neighboring areas to visit.

v. Medicinal Seed Villages:
   Two medicinal seed villages were established in Baragaon Okhlana and Panihavar in district Aligarh.

vi. Vermicompost Units:
   In order to encourage organic farming of medicinal crops, farmers were skilled to manufacture their own vermicompost in villages, using own resources.

1.13 Conclusion

Given the current trends, policy support, and demonstrated farmer interest, the rationale for promoting medicinal crop cultivation is stronger than ever. Western Uttar Pradesh, with its favorable agro-climatic conditions, established training infrastructure, and history of pilot success, stands ready to lead this transition. The initiative described in this book serves as a replicable model for mainstreaming medicinal agriculture across India.

CHAPTER 2

IDENTIFICATION AND SELECTION OF MEDICINAL SPECIES FOR FIELD-SCALE CULTIVATION

2.1 Medicinal Plants Used in Indian Systems of Medicine (ISM) and Homeopathy

India is home to one of the world's richest repositories of medicinal plants, many of which have been integral to its traditional healthcare systems for centuries. The Indian Systems of Medicine—comprising Ayurveda, Unani, Siddha, and Homeopathy—depend heavily on plant-based raw materials.

As per established literature, over 7,000 species of plants are used in Ayurveda, approximately 700 in Unani medicine, 600 in Siddha, 450 in Homeopathy, and about 30 species in Modern Allopathic medicine. However, the Ministry of AYUSH and other official institutions have standardized the use of about 1,500 medicinal plant species across these systems, with around 500 species commonly used for large-scale pharmaceutical preparations.

2.2 Species Widely Utilized by the ISM & H Industry

A study commissioned by the Department of Indian Systems of Medicine & Homeopathy (2000–2001) identified 162 medicinal plant species as core components in the formulation of traditional Indian medicines. These species account for approximately 71% of the total plant materials used in ISM & H manufacturing.

According to the Centre for Research, Planning, and Action (CERPA) report (2000-2001), nearly 198,054.71 metric tons of raw medicinal produce were consumed domestically by ISM & H industries during 1999–2000. Of this, 120,816.80 metric tons were drawn from just the aforementioned 162 species, underlining the critical dependency on wild-harvested raw material.

This over-reliance on wild collection has led to the rapid depletion of many species. Unsustainable harvesting practices not only threaten biodiversity but also undermine the availability of vital medicinal resources for future generations. Therefore, promoting the **field-scale cultivation** of medicinal plants is both a conservation imperative and an economic opportunity. This approach ensures a reliable supply of high-quality raw material, supports conservation efforts, and offers a viable livelihood avenue for farmers.

2.3 Selection of Medicinal Species for Cultivation in Western Uttar Pradesh

The concept of medicinal plant cultivation was relatively novel among the farming communities in Western Uttar Pradesh. Introducing new crops required a methodical approach to selecting species that were not only commercially viable but also agronomically suitable for the region's agro-climatic conditions.

A comprehensive literature review was undertaken to identify suitable species. Key reference documents included:

- *Cultivation Practices of Some Commercially Important Medicinal Plants* (NMPB, 2002) – 32 species
- *Report of the Task Force on Conservation and Sustainable Use of Medicinal Plants* (Planning Commission, 2000) – 25 species
- *Herbal Products: Current Status, Vision and Action Plan* (Report of the SAC-C, 2000) – 45 species

- *Demand Study for Selected Medicinal Plants* (Ministry of Health & Family Welfare, 2000–2001) – 162 species

These sources offered insight into species demand, cultivation practices, and conservation priorities.

Criteria for Selection

The final selection was guided by the following factors:

- High market demand from ISM & H pharmaceutical industries
- Adaptability to the agro-climatic conditions of Western Uttar Pradesh
- Ease of cultivation and post-harvest handling
- Availability of quality planting material
- Assured marketability at remunerative prices
- Cost-effective production potential

2.4 Preliminary Selection: 23 Medicinal Species

An initial list of 23 medicinal plant species was identified for cultivation trials (Table 2.1). For each species, detailed literature was developed in Hindi, the local language, to ensure accessibility for farmers. These were disseminated during awareness campaigns, training sessions, and farmer meets.

Table 2.1: Medicinal Plant Species Initially Identified for Cultivation

S.No.	Common Name	Botanical Name
1	Ashwagandha	*Withania somnifera* (L.) Dunal
2	Kalmegh	*Andrographis paniculata* Wall. ex Nees
3	Shatavari	*Asparagus racemosus* Willd
4	Mushkdana	*Abelmoschus moschatus* Medic
5	Jatropha	*Jatropha curcas* Linn.
6	Kaunch	*Mucuna pruriens* (Linn.) DC
7	Kanta Karanj	*Caesalpinia bonduc* (Linn.) Roxb.
8	Tulsi	*Ocimum sanctum* Linn.
9	Sanai	*Cassia angustifolia* Vahl.
10	Safed Musli	*Chlorophytum borivilianum* Sant & Fern.

S.No.	Common Name	Botanical Name
11	Amla	*Emblica officinalis* Gaertn.
12	Semal Musli	*Bombax ceiba* Linn.
13	Isabgol	*Plantago ovata* Forsk.
14	Mulethi	*Glycyrrhiza glabra* L.
15	Sarpgandha	*Rauvolfia serpentina* (L.) Benth. ex Kurz
16	Sadabahar	*Catharanthus roseus* (L.) G. Don.
17	Kuchla	*Strychnos nux-vomica* L.
18	Babchi	*Psoralea corylifolia* L.
19	Gwarpatha	*Aloe barbadensis* Mill.
20	Milk Thistle	*Silybum marianum* (L.) Gaertn.
21	Gulnar Farsi	*Punica granatum* L. (abortive variety)
22	Atrilal	*Ammi majus* L.
23	Stevia	*Stevia rebaudiana* Bertoni.

2.5 Final Selection: 12 Priority Species for Field-Scale Cultivation

Based on cultivation trials, market response, farmer feedback, and economic viability, 12 species emerged as most suitable for large-scale farming. These species demonstrated high market demand, good returns on investment, and compatibility with local conditions (Table 2.2).

Table 2.2: Priority Medicinal Species Recommended for Cultivation in Western Uttar Pradesh

S.No.	Botanical Name	Estimated Annual Demand (India)	Annual Growth Rate (%)
1	*Withania somnifera* (L.) Dunal	9,127.5 tons	9.1
2	*Andrographis paniculata* (Burm.f.) Wall. ex Nees.	2,197.3 tons	3.1
3	*Asparagus racemosus* Willd.	16,615 tons	15.1
4	*Cassia angustifolia* Vahl.	9,828 tons	21.8
5	*Emblica officinalis* Gaertn.	34,568.8 tons	22.5
6	*Mucuna pruriens* (L.) DC.	1,136.2 tons	17.5
7	*Ocimum sanctum* Linn.	5,014 tons	179

S.No.	Botanical Name	Estimated Annual Demand (India)	Annual Growth Rate (%)
8	*Rauvolfia serpentina* (L.) Benth. ex Kurz.	588.7 tons	11.6
9	*Caesalpinia bonduc* (L.) Roxb.	22.1 tons	13.2
10	*Chlorophytum borivilianum* Sant & Fern.	Data not available	—
11	*Aloe barbadensis* Mill.	2,389.6 tons	3.0
12	*Abelmoschus moschatus* Medik	1,887 tons	5.0

Source: Report – Demand Study for Selected Medicinal Plants (2000-2001)

These priority crops not only represent high-growth market opportunities but also offer a sustainable alternative to wild harvesting, enabling farmers in Western Uttar Pradesh to diversify their incomes and contribute to national herbal industry needs.

CHAPTER 3

DEMAND ESTIMATES FOR MEDICINAL PLANTS RAW PRODUCE

3.1 Estimating Demand for Medicinal Plant-Based Raw Materials in the Indian Pharmaceutical Industry

The estimation of demand for medicinal plant-based raw materials in India's pharmaceutical sector—especially in the Indian Systems of Medicine and Homeopathy (ISM&H)—is largely based on approximation rather than systematic studies. Currently, about **1.5 million practitioners** are engaged in using medicinal plants for both therapeutic and preventive healthcare in India.

According to the Ministry of AYUSH, 755,780 registered practitioners are involved in ISM&H therapies, supported by 7,843 ISM pharmacies and 851 homeopathic pharmacies, all contributing to the growing demand for herbal raw materials. However, the supply base for medicinal plants is under increasing stress due to a sharp global rise in demand for botanical raw materials used in herbal medicines and nutraceuticals.

Despite this growing demand, India lacks reliable demand-supply projections and systematic planning for the cultivation and conservation of medicinal plants. To date, only a few comprehensive studies—such as the CERPA Report (2000-2001) and Ved and Goraya (2008)—have attempted to quantify this demand. No major studies have been reported since then that provide updated and authentic data on the demand estimates of medicinal plant raw materials for ISM&H pharmaceutical industries.

3.2 Highlights of the CERPA Report (2000-2001)

The CERPA study, commissioned by the Department of ISM&H, Ministry of AYUSH, highlighted that over 1,200 medicinal plant species are in use or trade across India. Of these, 162 species have been identified as critically important, contributing to over 61% of total quantity used and 71% of forest-derived raw material supply.

Table 3.2: Estimated domestic demand for selected medicinal plants: Top 20 medicinal plants quantity- wise (CERPA Report 2000-2001):

Botanical name	Common name	1999-2000	
		Qty (tons)	Percent share (%)
Emblica officinalis Gaertn	Amla	15146.7	12.5
Asparagus racemosus Willd	Shatavari	8246.3	6.8
Withania somnifera (Linn.) Dunal	Ashwagandha	5905.1	4.9
Terminalia chebula Retz.	Harar/Halela Zard	5413.4	4.5
Saraca asoca (*Roxb.*) *de Wilde*	Ashok	5331.8	4.4
Aegle marmelos (Linn.) Correa *ex. Roxb.*	Bel	4479.8	3.7
Cassia angustifolia Vahl.	Sanai/ Sonapatri	4356.2	3.6
Adhatoda vasica Nees	Adusa/Arusa	4211.9	3.5
Piper longum Linn.	Pippali, Filfildaraz	2951.8	2.4
Bacopa monnieri (Linn.) Pennell	Brahmi	2650.1	2.2
Sida cordifolia Linn.	Kanghi	2677.8	2.2
Ocimum sanctum Linn.	Tulsi	2371.7	2.0
Bambusa bambos Druce.	Vansalochan/Tabasheer	2153.5	1.8
Boerhaavia diffusa Linn.	Punarnava	2182.3	1.8
Azadirachta indica A. Juss.	Neem	2039.3	1.7
Solanum nigrum Linn.	Makoya/ Inab-US-Salab	2005.1	1.7
Weodfordia fructicosa Kurz.	Dhataki, Dhai	2014.3	1.7
Andrographis paniculata Nees	Kalmegh	1886.2	1.6
Syzygium aromaticum L.	Long/lavang.	1967.8	1.6
Tinospora cordifolia (Wild)	Giloe, Guudchi	1897.3	1.6

Table 3.3: Estimated domestic demand for selected medicinal plants by value:

Botanical name	Common name	1999-2000	
		Value (Rs. Lakhs)	Percent share (%)
Bambusa bambos Druce.	Vansalochan/Tabasheer	6460.5	9.6
Emblica officinalis Gaertn	Amla	6058.7	9.0
Syzygium aromaticum Linn	Long/lavang.	5903.4	8.8
Asparagus racemosus Willd	Shatavari	5772.4	8.6
Piper longum Linn.	Pippali, Filfildaraz	4427.7	6.6
Withania somnifera (Linn.) Dunal	Ashwagandha	3543.1	5.3
Aconitum heterophyllum Wall ex Royale	Ativisha/Atis	2505.1	3.7
Swertia chirata Buch. Ham.	Chirayata	2393.1	3.6
Cuminum cyminum Linn	Zeera/ Zeera safaid	1652.0	2.5
Saraca asoca (*Roxb.*) de Willde	Ashok	1599.5	2.4
Cassia angustifolia Vahl.	Sanai/ Sonapatri	1306.9	1.9
Commiphora wightii (Arn.) Bhandari	Guggal	1059.2	1.6
Aegle marmelos (Linn.) Correa *ex. Roxb.*	Bel	896.0	1.3
Anacyclus pyrethrum DC.	Aquarqarha	903.0	1.3
Gentiana kurroo Royle.	Kuru	884.7	1.3
Nardostachys jatamansi DC.	Jatamansi/ Sumbul ut Teeb	856.8	1.3
Bacopa monnieri (Linn.) Pennell	Brahmi	795.0	1.2
Piper cubeba Linn. F.	Kababchini	743.6	1.1
Aloe barbadensis Mill.	Gheekwar, Elva Musabbar	650.8	1.0
Boerhaavia diffusa Linn.	Punarnava	654.7	1.0

Table 3.4 : List of 162 medicinal plants widely used in the Indian Systems of Medicine & Homeopathy

S.NO.	Botanical Name
1	*Abies webbiana* Lindl
2	*Achillea millefolium* Linn
3	*Achyranthus aspera* Linn.
4	*Aconitum chasmanthum* (Stapf. Ex. Volmes)
5	*Aconitum heterophyllum* Wallich ex Royla
6	*Acorus calamus* Linn.
7	*Adhatoda vasica* Nees.
8	*Aegle marmelos* (L.) Corr. Ex. Schultz.
9	*Albizzia lebbeck* (L.) Benth.
10	*Aletris farmosa* Linn.
11	*Aloe barbadensis* Mill.
12	*Alstonia scholaris* (L.) Br.
13	*Althaea officinalis* Linn.
14	*Anacyclus pyrethrum* DC.
15	*Andrographis paniculata* (Burm. F.) Wall.
16	*Anethum sowa* Kurz.
17	*Aquilaria agallocha* Roxb.
18	*Aralia racemosa* Linn.
19	*Arnicaa montana* Linn.
20	*Artemisia absinthium* L.
21	*Asparagus racemosus* Willd.
22	*Azadirachta indica* A. Juss.
23	*Bacopa monnieri* (L.)Penn.
24	*Baliospermum montanum* Muell-Arg.
25	*Bambusa bamboo* Druce
26	*Baptisia tinctoria* R.Br.
27	*Berberis aristata* DC.
28	*Boerhaavia diffusa* Linn.
29	*Bryonia alba* Linn.
30	*Butea monosperma* (Lamk.) Taub
31	*Caesalpinia sappan* Linn.
32	*Calandula officinalis* Linn.
33	*Callicarpa macrophylla* Vahl.
34	*Carduss marianus* Linn.
35	*Carum carvi* Linn.
36	*Cassia angustifolia* Vahl.
37	*Cassia fistula* Linn.
38	*Ceanothus americanus* Linn.
39	*Celastrus paniculatus* Willd.
40	*Centaurea behen* Linn.
41	*Centella asiatica* (Linn.) Urban
42	*Chelidonium majus* Linn.
43	*Cinnamomum tamala* Nees & Eberm
44	*Cinnamomum zeylanicum* Nees
45	*Cissampelos pareira* Linn.
46	*Clerodendrum phlomoidis* L.f.
47	*Clerodendrum serratum* (L.) Moon
48	*Coleus uettiveroides* K.C.Jacab
49	*Commiphora wightii* (Arn.) Bhandari
50	*Convolvalus pluricaulis* Choisy
51	*Convolvulus scammonia* Linn.
52	*Coscinium fenestratum* Colebr
53	*Crataeva nurvala* Buch-Ham
54	*Cryptolepis buchanani* Roem & Schult
55	*Cuminum cyminum* L.
56	*Curculigo orchioides* Gaertn.
57	*Curcuma zedoaria* Roxb.

S.NO.	Botanical Name
58	*Cyperus rotundus* Linn.
59	*Datura metel* Linn.
60	*Desmodium gangeticum* (L.) DC.
61	*Doronicum hookeri* hook. f.
62	*Elaeocarpus ganitrus* Roxb.
63	*Embelia ribes* Burm. f
64	*Embilica officinalis* Gaertn.
65	*Ephedra gerardiana* Wall.
66	*Euphrasia officinalis* Linn.
67	*Fumaria parviflora* Lam.
68	*Garcinia indica* Choisy
69	*Gelsemium sempervirens* Ait
70	*Gentiana kurroo* Royle
71	*Gloriosa superba* Linn
72	*Glycyrrhiza glabra* Linn.
73	*Gmelina arborea* Roxb.
74	*Gymnema sylvestre* (Rety.) R.Br.
75	*Habenaria intermedia* D. Don.
76	*Hemidesmus indicus* (L.) R.Br.
77	*Holarrhena antidysenterica* Wall.
78	*Hydrastis canadensis* Linn.
79	*Hypericum perforatum* Linn.
80	*Ipomoea petaloidea* Choisy
81	*Inula racemosa* Hook. f.
82	*Lavandula stoechas* Linn.
83	*Ledum palustre* Linn.
84	*Lobelia inflata* linn.
85	*Madhuca indica* J.F.
86	*Mallotus philippinensis* Muell. Arg.
87	*Malva sylvestris* Linn.
88	*Mesua ferrea* Linn.
89	*Microstylis wallichii* Lindl
90	*Mucuna prurita* Hook
91	*Nardostachys jatamansi* DC.
92	*Ocimum sanctum* Linn.
93	*Oenanthe crocata* Linn.
94	*Onosma bracteatum* Wall.
95	*Onosma echioldes* Linn.
96	*Operculina turpethum* (L.) Silva Manso
97	*Oroxylum indicum* Vent.
98	*Paederia foetida* Linn.
99	*Paeonia officinalis* Linn.
100	*Parreira brava* (abutua)
101	*Passiflora incarnata* Linn.
102	*Peristrophe bicalyculata* Nees
103	*Phyllanthus niruri* Linn.
104	*Phytolacca americana* Linn.
105	*Picrorhiza kurrooa* Royle ex Benth
106	*Pilocarpus jaborandi* (Pilocarpus microphyllus Stapf ex Wardleworthy)
107	*Piper chaba* Hunter
108	*Piper cubeca* Linn. f.
109	*Piper longum* Linn.
110	*Pistacia integerrima* Stewart
111	*Pistacia lentiscus* Linn.
112	*Pluchea lanceolata* Oliver & Hiern.
113	*Plumbago zeylanica* Linn.
114	*Polygonatum cirrhifolium* (Wall.) Royle
115	*Prunus cerasoides* D. Don.
116	*Pterocarpus santalinus* Linn. f.
117	*Krameria triandra* Ruiz and Pavon
118	*Rauvolfia serpentina* (L.) Benth. Ex Kurz.
119	*Rhus parviflora* Roxb.
120	*Rhus toxicodendron* Linn.
121	*Rosa damascena* Mill

S.NO.	Botanical Name
122	*Rubia cordifolia* Linn.
123	*Sabal serrulata* Schult
124	*Salmalia malabarica* Schott & Endl
125	*Salvia haematodes* Linn.
126	*Santalaum album* Linn.
127	*Saussurea hypoleuca* spreng
128	*Saussurea Costus* (Falc.) Lipsch.
129	*Saraca asoca* (roxb.) DC. Willd.
130	*Scindapsus officinalis* (Roxb.) Schott.
131	*Shorea robusta* Gaertn. f.
132	*Sida cordifolia* Linn.
133	*Sida rhombifolia* Linn.
134	*Sisymbrium irio* Linn.
135	*Smilax china* Linn.
136	*Solanum indicum* Linn.
137	*Solanum nigrum* Linn.
138	*Sphaeranthus indicus* Linn.
139	*Strychnos nux-vomica* Linn.
140	*Swertia chirata* Buch. Ham.
141	*Symplocos racemosa* Roxb.
142	*Syzygium aromaticum* (L.) Merr. & L.M. Perry
143	*Terminalia arjuna* W. & A.

S.NO.	Botanical Name
144	*Terminalia chebula* Retz.
145	*Thuja occidentalis* Linn.
146	*Tinospora cordifolia* (Willd.) Miers.
147	*Trachyspermum ammi* (L.) Sprague
148	*Trachyspermum roxburghianum* (DC) Sprag
149	*Tribulus terrestris* Linn.
150	*Trichosanthes dioica* Roxb.
151	*Trigonella foenum-graecum* Linn.
152	*Tylophora indica* (Burm.f.) Merr.
153	*Uraia picta* (Jacq.) Desv.
154	*Urtica uens* Henn.
155	*Valeriana wallichii* DC.
156	*Vernonia cineria* (L.) Less.
157	*Vetiveria zizanioides* (Linn.) Nash.
158	*Vitex negundo* Linn.
159	*Withania somnifera* (L.) Dunal.
160	*Woodfordia fruticosa* Kurtz.
161	*Zanthoxylum armatum* DC.
162	*Zizyphus sativa* Gaertn.

Source: (CERPA Report 2000-2001)

Table 1 & 2 displays data for the high demand top 20 plants by quantity and value. It is evident that 66.2 percent of the demand for the raw materials of 162 medicinal plants is met by these 20 plants which collectively represent 73.1% of the entire value.

3.3 Demand Estimates of Botanical Raw Drugs (Ved & Goraya, 2007)

Ved and Goraya's landmark survey remains one of the most authoritative snapshots of India's medicinal-plant economy:

- Scale of the manufacturing base. In 2005–06 India hosted roughly 9,500 registered herbal-product manufacturers, alongside a large but unquantified constellation of cottage-scale, unregistered units.
- Diversity in trade. The authors documented 960 medicinal plant species supplying 1,289 distinct botanical raw drugs to domestic markets.
- Heavy-demand species. Only 178 species recorded annual off-take above 100 t, yet these few species accounted for ≈ 80 % of total industrial demand, underscoring a pronounced concentration in raw-material use.
- Aggregate demand and value. National consumption of botanical raw materials was estimated at 319,500 t, valued at about INR 1,069 crore (≈ USD 240 million) for 2005–06.
- Sector turnover. Total turnover of the herbal industry was placed at INR 8,800 crore (≈ USD 2 billion) for the same period.
- Documented supply. Data gathered from state agencies suggested an annual domestic production of only ~120,000 t, highlighting a substantial supply–demand gap.
- Data gaps. No national-level, species-wise cultivation statistics were available, revealing the sector's continuing informality and the urgent need for systematic monitoring.

Together with the FRLHT–UNDP demand study (Section 3.3.2), Ved and Goraya's analysis provides a rare, quantitative baseline. Nonetheless, the medicinal-plant supply chain remains largely unorganised; definitive figures on production, trade flows, and cultivation area are still lacking and represent a priority research frontier.

3.4 Export–Import Dynamics of Medicinal Plant Raw Produce*

According to the Ministry of AYUSH (2024), the herbal raw material market in India has witnessed exponential growth, expanding from USD 2.85 billion in 2014 to USD 23.4 billion in 2023. During this period, exports doubled—rising from USD 1.09 billion to USD 2.16 billion—firmly positioning India as a global leader in traditional medicine.

A market study by Exim Bank reports that 880 medicinal plant species are actively traded, both within domestic markets and internationally. Of these, 42 species are primarily imported, while 48 species are exported. Notably, China dominates the global herbal trade with approximately 30% share by value, followed by South Korea, the United States, India, and Chile. In the Asian context, Singapore and Hong Kong emerge as significant re-exporters of medicinal botanicals.

Within India, the domestic traditional medicine sector consumes more than 177,000 metric tons of raw medicinal plant material annually, valued at around INR 627.90 crore. It is estimated that the total commercial turnover associated with medicinal plant trade in India approaches USD 1 billion annually. In fiscal year 2023, India exported Ayurvedic herbal products worth approximately USD 628 million. Since 2015, export values have risen steadily, with a temporary decline in 2020–21 (USD 246.78 million) due to global disruptions. However, the sector rebounded strongly, and total AYUSH exports reached USD 1.09 billion (INR 9,000 crore) by 2023.

The Annual Report (2022–23) of the Department of Commerce, Government of India highlights that the country's pharmaceutical exports during 2020–21 stood at INR 1,46,260 crore, while imports were INR 42,943 crore. Maharashtra led the nation in export performance, registering its highest-ever export value of USD 447.46 million in FY 2022–23, reflecting a 6.03% growth over the previous year.

Among individual herbal products, Psyllium Husk (Isabgol) stands out as India's most valuable export item in the medicinal plant category, contributing to nearly 70% of the total export value of the country's herbal produce.

These trends indicate a strong potential for India's herbal drug export market to scale up to USD 10 billion by 2030, especially with enhanced integration in global supply chains, better marketing, and focused value addition.

Given India's diverse agroclimatic zones, there exists a unique opportunity to scale up field-level cultivation of high-demand medicinal crops. Such an expansion would not only meet rising domestic demand but also open significant export avenues. Strategically promoting medicinal crop farming across suitable regions in India can lead to a robust rural economy, empower farmers, and contribute to sustainable agricultural growth.

**The information on trade aspects of medicinal plants ,including marketing, exports, and imports are based on a comprehensive review of existing literature including government reports, AYUSH resources, and other relevant sources. Nevertheless, author does not owe any responsibility for their accuracy.*

Source:

1. *Growth Potential of AYUSH in India – Invest India (July 10, 2020).*
2. *AYUSH and Herbal Products exports Register 3.6% Growth in 2023-24. WWW. Pharmabiz.com*
3. *Directorate General of Commercial Intelligence and Statistics (DGCI & S), Government of India, New Delhi*

3.5 Conclusion and Gaps

The above two studies—CERPA (2000-2001) and Ved & Goraya (2008)—remain the most authoritative sources of information on the demand and supply of medicinal plant raw materials in India. However, the sector continues to suffer from:

- A lack of updated and reliable data
- An unorganized production and distribution framework
- Poor coordination between cultivation, conservation, and market demand

To truly harness the economic and healthcare potential of medicinal crops, India must undertake systematic, updated research on demand projections, region-wise cultivation data, and supply chain dynamics of medicinal plants used in ISM&H.

CHAPTER 4

DOCUMENTATION OF LITERATURE ON CULTIVATION AND MARKETING OF MEDICINAL CROPS

This chapter presents a comprehensive overview of the initiatives undertaken to promote awareness and knowledge about the cultivation and marketing of medicinal crops among farmers in Western Uttar Pradesh, India. Recognizing the significant potential of medicinal crop farming in improving rural livelihoods, strategic efforts were made to document best practices and disseminate relevant information to the farming community.

Special emphasis was placed on selecting medicinal plant species that are commercially viable, agronomically feasible, cost-effective, and in high demand. As part of this foundational effort, extensive documentation was undertaken on agrotechniques, post-harvest storage, and marketing avenues. This initiative culminated in the development of model pamphlets, farmer-friendly booklets, and a marketing directory—all designed to support informed decision-making and encourage widespread adoption of medicinal crop farming.

4.1 Development of Model Pamphlets on Selected Medicinal Species

To facilitate grassroots adoption and awareness, full-color, field-level pamphlets were developed for 23 medicinal plant species prioritized for their economic and therapeutic value. These pamphlets were distributed free of cost to interested farmers and stakeholders.

A Sneak Peek at the Medicinal Crop Pamphlet(s):

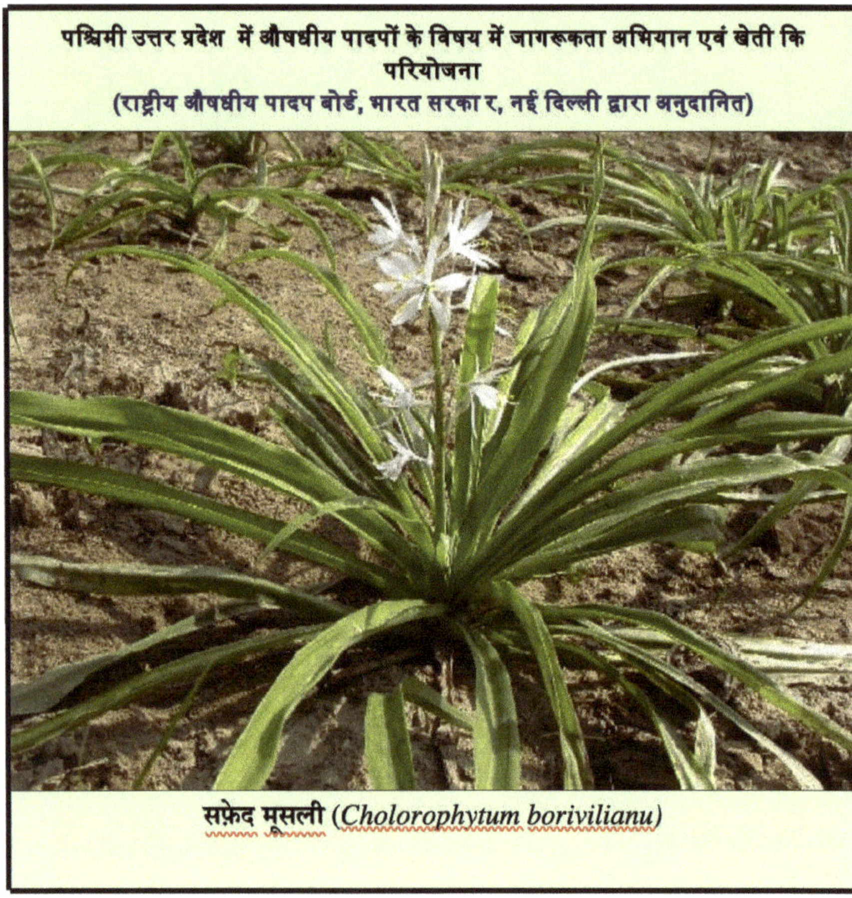
पश्चिमी उत्तर प्रदेश में औषधीय पादपों के विषय में जागरूकता अभियान एवं खेती कि परियोजना
(राष्ट्रीय औषधीय पादप बोर्ड, भारत सरका र, नई दिल्ली द्वारा अनुदानित)
सफ़ेद मूसली (Cholorophytum borivilianu)

Visuals of selected informational pamphlets on medicinal crops, covering agrotechniques and marketing, distributed to farmers at the programs' inception to support informed cultivation practices-

Each pamphlet covered the following:

- Scientific, Hindi, and common names
- Historical significance and medicinal applications
- Cultivation guidelines, including:

- Soil and land preparation
- Propagation techniques
- Nutrient management and fertilizer application
- Irrigation schedules
- Weeding, harvesting, and collection methods
- Post-harvest processing and storage
- Estimated yields and plant parts used

4.1 List of Medicinal Plants Covered:

1. *Emblica officinalis* (Amla)
2. *Catharanthus roseus* (Sadabahar)
3. *Jatropha curcas* (Jatropha)
4. *Glycyrrhiza glabra* (Mulethi)
5. *Bombax ceiba* (Semal Musli)
6. *Andrographis paniculata* (Kalmegh)
7. *Cassia angustifolia* (Sanai)
8. *Rauvolfia serpentina* (Sarpgandha)
9. *Withania somnifera* (Ashwagandha)
10. *Mucuna pruriens* (Konch)
11. *Caesalpinia crista* (Kantakaranj)
12. *Punica granatum* (Gulnar farsi – abortive type)
13. *Abelmoschus moschatus* (Mushkdana)
14. *Asparagus racemosus* (Shatavari)
15. *Ocimum sanctum* (Tulsi)
16. *Plantago ovata* (Isabgol)
17. *Chlorophytum borivilianum* (Safed Musli)
18. *Aloe barbadensis* (Aloe vera)
19. *Stevia rebaudiana* (Stevia)
20. *Silybum marianum* – Milk Thistle (Doodhpatra Dudhi)
21. *Psoralea corylifolia* (Babchi)
22. *Ammi majus* (Atrilal)
23. *Aegle marmelos* (Bael)

Additionally, farmers received verbal and written guidance on necessary **precautions** before shifting from conventional to medicinal crop farming, helping them avoid common pitfalls.

4.2 Publication of a Farmer-Friendly Booklet in Hindi

To further strengthen outreach efforts, a comprehensive **Hindi-language booklet** titled **"पश्चिमी उत्तर प्रदेश में औषधीय फसलों की खेती—संभावनाएं और विकास"** was published. This booklet was well received and proved instrumental in training and awareness campaigns.

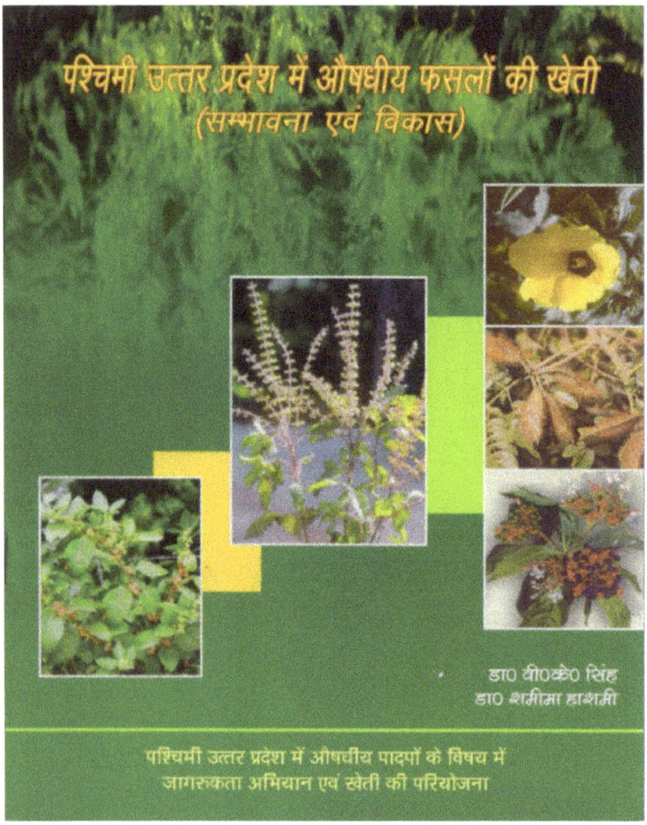

Fig 4.3 Farmers' Booklet: A Guide to Cultivating High-Demand Medicinal Crops Agrotechniques and Market Potential in Western U.P.

Key Contents of the Booklet:

1. The necessity of medicinal crop cultivation in Uttar Pradesh
2. Global market outlook for medicinal plant products
3. Overview of awareness and training programs in Western Uttar Pradesh
4. Multi-tier cultivation approaches

5. Recommended trees and shrubs for village-level plantations
6. Safety and preparatory measures for new medicinal farmers
7. Agrotechniques for selected species, including:
   - *Amla, Kalmegh, Kantakaranj, Isabgol, Sadabahar, Sanai, Gulnar farsi, Safed Musli, Jatropha, Sarpgandha, Mushkdana, Aloe vera, Mulethi, Ashwagandha, Shatavari, Semal Musli, Konch,* and *Tulsi*
8. Economics of cultivation: Cost–benefit analysis
9. Post-harvest handling and storage methods
10. Demand estimates for raw botanicals in India and abroad
11. Government guidelines and prioritized species for cultivation
12. Directory of 33 national research centers working on medicinal crops
13. Contact details of major pharmaceutical companies, traders, and exporters in Ayurveda, Unani, Siddha, and Homoeopathy sectors
14. Disease management and integrated pest control measures, including recommended fungicides and insecticides

4.3 Compilation of a Marketing Directory for Medicinal Produce

A dedicated **Marketing Directory** was created to help farmers establish direct linkages with legitimate buyers and ensure fair pricing. This publication became a cornerstone for commercial success and market penetration.

Contents of the Directory:

- Contact details of over 2,100 manufacturers, traders, and suppliers from 63 districts in Uttar Pradesh and Uttarakhand
- Information on:
  - Current supply chain dynamics and pricing trends
  - Major procurement centers for medicinal raw drugs across India
  - Market channels and distribution systems
  - WHO-guided Good Agricultural and Collection Practices (GACP)

4.4 Challenges in Marketing Medicinal Produce

Despite substantial progress in cultivation practices and farmer participation, marketing remained a persistent challenge. Farmers encountered difficulties in monetizing their harvests due to:

- Lack of assured buy-back agreements from pharmaceutical firms
- Fragmented and unregulated market structures
- Absence of a price assurance mechanism backed by the government

Even after over two decades since its establishment, the National Medicinal Plants Board (NMPB) under the Ministry of AYUSH has not succeeded in building a robust, organized, and farmer-centric marketing infrastructure. This remains a critical policy and implementation gap, hindering the growth of small and marginal farmers engaged in medicinal crop production.

CHAPTER 5

PROVIDING QUALITY PLANTING MATERIALS OF MEDICINAL CROPS TO FARMERS

Medicinal crop farming is a relatively new concept for most Indian farmers. Unlike traditional cereal and food crops, the planting materials for medicinal plants are not readily available in the open market. Although the medicinal plant sector has seen significant growth in recent years, the supply of quality planting material remains a major challenge. Nevertheless, certain organizations—particularly in states such as Rajasthan, Madhya Pradesh, Maharashtra, and Uttarakhand—have begun supplying planting materials of selected medicinal crops.

5.1 Non-Availability of Quality Planting Materials for High-Value Medicinal Crops

One of the major constraints faced by farmers is the lack of reliable and high-quality planting materials. Much of what is currently available is of substandard quality, resulting in poor crop performance and low yields. As a result, many medicinal plant species with significant market demand and therapeutic potential are yet to be cultivated on a commercial scale.

This situation has deprived progressive farmers of the opportunity to diversify their income through medicinal crop cultivation. To address this, farmers were encouraged to raise their own planting materials locally, thus ensuring better control over quality and sustainability in future crop cycles.

5.2 Need for Genetically Upgraded Planting Materials

The availability of genetically superior planting material is essential for the success of medicinal crop farming. Many farmers have experienced frustration due to poor plant performance resulting from inferior or non-authenticated seeds and saplings. To ensure consistent and standard production of raw materials for pharmaceutical industries, agricultural research institutions must prioritize the development and distribution of improved planting materials.

5.3 Project Initiative: Distribution of Quality Planting Material

As part of the project's efforts to promote medicinal farming in rural areas, quality seeds of high-demand medicinal crops were procured from recognized centers in Rajasthan and Madhya Pradesh and distributed to farmers across Western Uttar Pradesh. The distribution was made available at subsidized rates, enabling farmers to initiate cultivation with minimal investment (Table 5.1)

Details of Quality Seed Distribution to Farmers

Table 5.1

S. No.	Name of Medicinal Plant	Quantity Distributed	Number of Farmers Benefited
1.	Ashwagandha	37 Kg	29
2.	Sonamukhi	40 Kg	35
3.	Kaunch	20 Kg	25
4.	Jatropha	20 Kg	27
5.	Mushkdana	20 Kg	30
6.	Kalmegh	05 Kg	30
7.	Kanta Karanj	10 Kg	08
8.	Isabgol	10 Kg	03
9.	Chandrashoor	05 Kg	05
	Total	**167 Kg**	**192**

This initiative benefited 192 farmers, providing a solid foundation for promoting medicinal crop cultivation in the region.

5.4 Advanced Training for Farmers Outside Uttar Pradesh

In order to build capacity and provide **hands-on expertise** to farmers and prospective growers, two specialized training programs were conducted at the **Rajasthan Agro Forestry Corporation, Jodhpur**. These programs trained **58 farmers** from various districts of Western Uttar Pradesh.

First Batch of Progressive Farmers' Training on Medicinal Crops Cultivation and Marketing

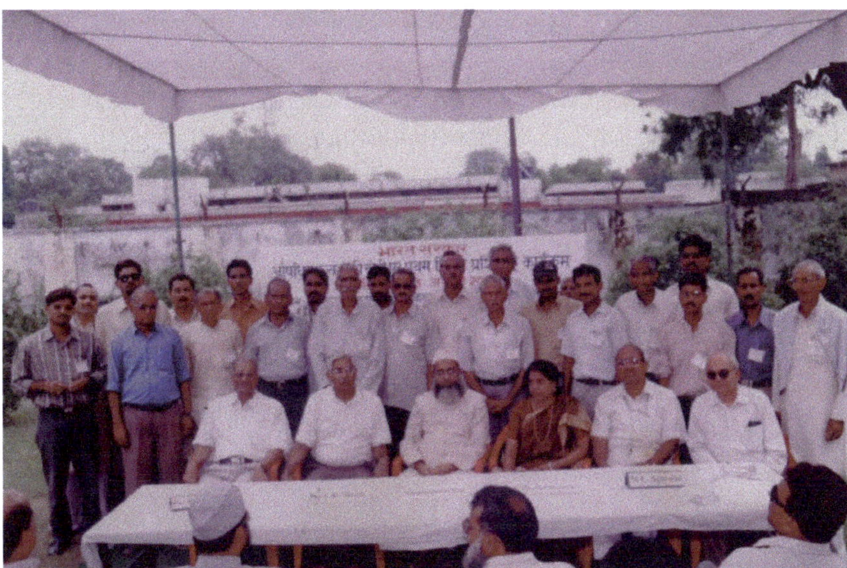

Fig 5.1 A Group Photograph of Progressive Farmers Proceeding to Rajasthan Agroforestry Corporation, Jodhpur for Advanced Training on Agrotechniques and Marketing of High-demand Medicinal Crops. Sitting on the Dais are: Mr. M.C. Agarwal, Regional Distributor, Mahendra Tractors, Aligarh, Dr. V.K. Singh, Project Director, Hakm Imran Ullaha Khan, Assistant Director, Mrs. Shamima Hashmi, Co-Principal Investigator, Dr. A.K. Tomar, Expert on Economics of Medicinal Produce, Dr. S.H. Afaq, Professor of Pharmacognosy (left to right).

Each training group was guided by project Agriculture Officer and participated under the leadership of Shri R.P.P. Singh, the Group Leader. To ensure identification and official recognition, Identity Cards were issued to all trainee farmers by the Project Office.

These training programs enabled farmers to:

- Learn scientifically proven cultivation practices
- Gain insights into market trends and buyer expectations
- Observe model farms and best practices in medicinal plant production

Conclusion

The availability of authentic and high-quality planting materials, coupled with technical training and institutional support, is vital for the success of medicinal crop farming in India. While the project took significant steps to address these foundational challenges, it also highlighted the need for continued institutional backing and research-driven support systems to ensure long-term sustainability and profitability for farmers entering this promising sector.

CHAPTER 6

DISSEMINATION OF INFORMATION

The success of any innovative agricultural initiative hinges on the effective dissemination of knowledge. Since medicinal crop cultivation was a relatively novel concept in Western Uttar Pradesh at the inception of this project, concerted efforts were made to raise awareness, educate farmers, and build robust institutional support mechanisms. A multi-dimensional strategy was adopted to ensure that farmers received timely, accurate, and accessible information through a range of outreach and support channels.

6.1 Establishment of Facilitation-cum-Information Center

To centralize the flow of information and services, a Facilitation-cum-Information Center was established at the Regional Research Institute of Unani Medicine (CCRUM), Government of India, in Aligarh. This center served as the operational nerve center for all project activities and played a pivotal role in farmer engagement, technical support, and capacity building.

Key Functions of the Center:

1. Operated as a one-stop facility for conservation, cultivation, and marketing support.
2. Maintained a comprehensive literature bank on agrotechnology and market trends for priority medicinal crops.

3. Distributed verified planting materials including seeds and cuttings.
4. Offered technical support across the cropping cycle—from land preparation to post-harvest storage.
5. Facilitated farmer-market linkages to ensure fair prices and profitable returns.
6. Convened Project Steering Committees, Farmer Interactions, and Buyer-Seller Meets to align stakeholders in the ISM&H (AYUSH) sector.
7. Oversaw demonstration plots in 35 villages, offering on-site practical guidance.
8. Assisted farmers and entrepreneurs in preparing detailed project proposals for financial support from the National Medicinal Plants Board (NMPB).
9. Compiled and published a Marketing Directory featuring details of traders, processors, and exporters.
10. Provided dedicated handholding support for first-time farmers entering medicinal crop cultivation.
11. Promoted sustainable practices by training farmers in vermitechnology and facilitating the establishment of vermicompost units.
12. Regularly updated stakeholders on the latest research and availability of elite planting material.

6.2 Organizing Farmer Meetings and Awareness Events

Recognizing the importance of grassroots-level engagement, a series of Farmer Awareness Meetings were organized. These forums facilitated knowledge-sharing, addressed local cultivation challenges, and fostered farmer-to-farmer learning.

Between 2002 and 2006, 14 major Farmers' Meets were organized across key rural blocks in Western Uttar Pradesh, including Aligarh, Hathras, Etah, and Firozabad. These gatherings provided valuable exposure to the cultivation and marketing of medicinal crops with demonstrable market demand.

Farmers' Meet Highlights: Agrotechniques and Marketing of Medicinal Crops in Western U.P.

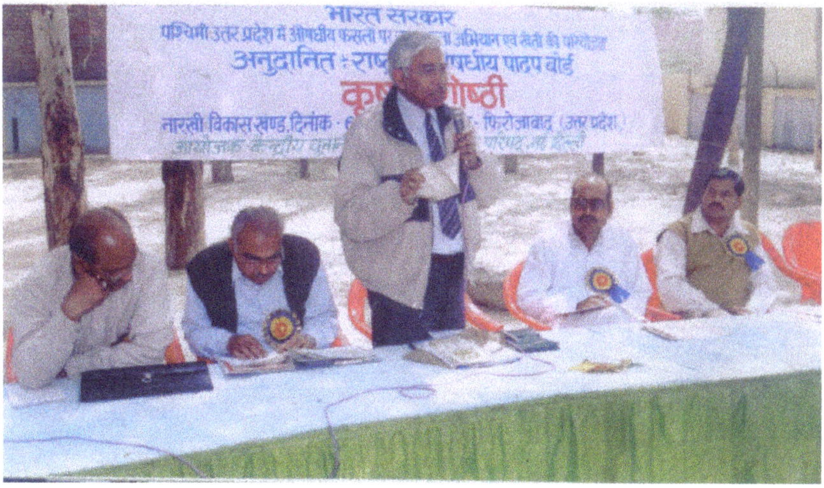

Fig 6.1: Farmers' Meet on Cultivation and Marketing in Progress: Dr. V.K. Singh, Project Director Addressing the Farmers on 6th May 2005 at Narkhi Development Block, District Firozabad, Explains Economic Benefits of Medicinal Crops Cultivation

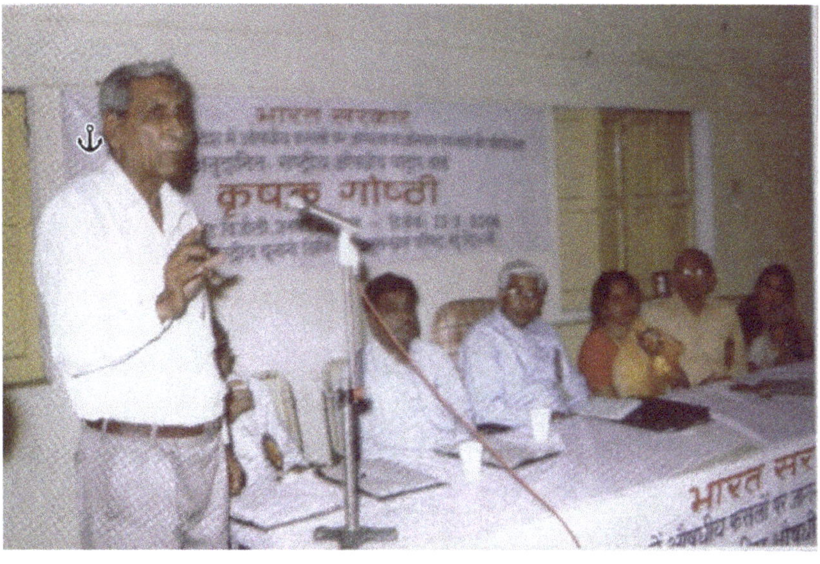

Fig 6.2:Mr. R.P.P Singh, Agriculture Officer Addressing the Farmers on Agrotechniques and Marketing of Medicinal Crops at Bijoli Development Block, District Aligarh on 23rd March 2006.

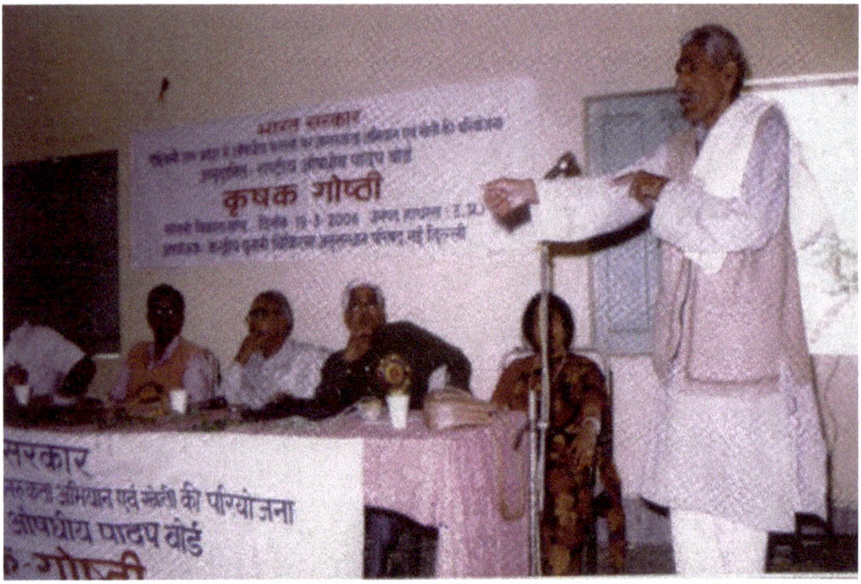

Fig 6.3 Shri Bhagwati Prasad, A Progressive Farmer Sharing his Experience of Cultivating Sanai (Cassia angustifolia) Medicinal Crop in his Field During the Farmers' Meet at Bijoli Development Block,District Aligarh

6.3 Farmers' Meets Conducted Under the Project

Table 6.1:

S. No.	Location (Development Block)	Date	Number of Participants
1	Jawan, Aligarh	18th August 2002	150
2	Gonda, Aligarh	15th September 2002	76
3	Atrauli, Aligarh	21st September 2009	82
4	Lodha, Aligarh	22nd December 2002	155
5	Dhanipur, Aligarh	29th December 2002	74
6	Sikandra Rao, Hathras	30th January 2005	110
7	Firozabad, Firozabad	1st March 2005	85
8	Narkhi, Firozabad	6th March 2005	78
9	Awagarh, Etah	16th March 2005	108
10	Jalesar, Etah	20th March 2005	110
11	Sadhu Ashram, Aligarh	27th November 2005	215
12	Sasni, Hathras	19th March 2006	70
13	Bijoli, Aligarh	23rd March 2006	140

Total Participation and Outcomes:

- Over 1,450 farmers attended these regional meets.
- Around 150 progressive farmers were selected for advanced training and supported in establishing demonstration plots.

6.4 Key Themes of Farmer Meetings

Each meeting was thematically structured and featured expert-led sessions that covered:

- Agrotechniques for the selected medicinal species.
- Economic feasibility and cost-benefit analysis.
- Post-harvest practices to ensure product quality and extended shelf-life.
- Integrated pest and disease management.
- Stepwise guidance for transitioning from traditional crops to medicinal farming systems.

Progressive farmers who had already adopted medicinal crops were invited to share their success stories, building trust and motivating fellow participants. An open question-and-answer session followed each expert presentation to address individual concerns and queries.

Participants were also given free literature on:

- Agronomic practices for 23 medicinal crops.
- Market trends and buyer directories.
- Disease identification charts and crop protection schedules.
- Verified sources for obtaining elite planting materials.

To reduce risk exposure, farmers were advised to start with small-scale trial plots before transitioning to full-scale medicinal crop cultivation based on field performance and profitability.

Importantly, these events were presided over by local Block Development Officers (BDOs), lending official credibility and administrative support to the initiative.

6.5 Centralized National Farmers' Meet

A landmark event—the Centralized Farmer Meet—was organized on 15th April 2003 at Aligarh. This high-level program was designed specifically for progressive farmers from the region and focused on advanced training, marketing strategies, and networking with stakeholders.

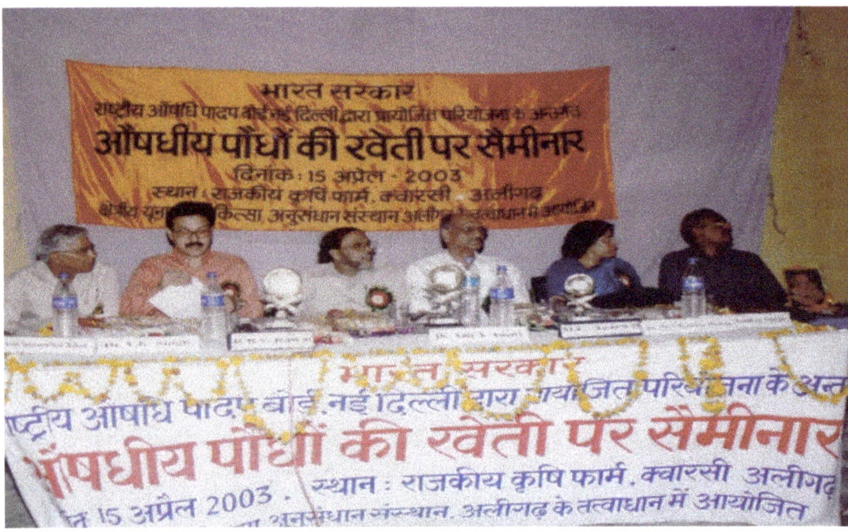
भारत सरकार
औषधीय पौधों की खेती पर सैमीनार
दिनांक : 15 अप्रैल - 2003

Fig 6.5 :A view of Inauguration Ceremony of National Farmers' Meet on Agro-techniques and Marketing of Medicinal Crops at Aligarh, held on 15th April 2003. Sitting on the Dais are Dr. V.K. Singh, Project Director, Dr. R.B.S. Rawat, former CEO, National Medicinal Plants Board, New Delhi, Dr. Anis Ahmad Ansari, Advisor, Department of ISM & H, Government of India, Mr. M.C. Agarwal, Regional Distributor, Mahendra Tractors, Aligarh, Mrs. Shamima Hashmi, Co-Principal Investigator, Mr. Ram Kripal Singh, Superintendent of Police (City), Aligarh (left to right).

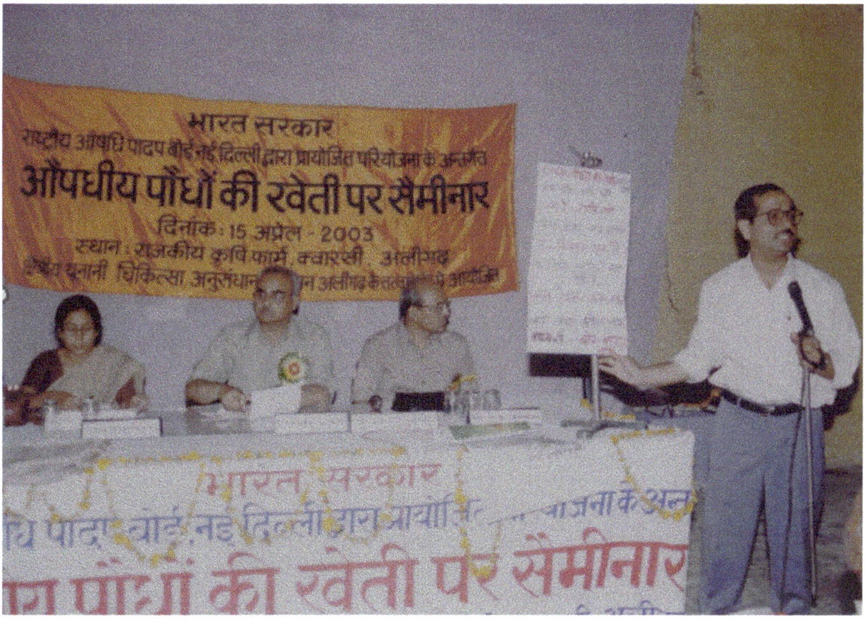
भारत सरकार
औषधीय पौधों की खेती पर सैमीनार
दिनांक : 15 अप्रैल - 2003

Fig 6.6 :Professor Shweta Yadav Chairing the Technical Session of National Meet on Agro-techniques and Marketing of Medicinal Crops at Aligarh. Sitting on the Dais are Dr. A.K.S. Chauhan and Dr. A.K. Tomar, Co-chairman (left to right).

Highlights of the Event:

- Expert presentations on high-demand species and market dynamics.
- Two technical sessions, followed by a panel discussion featuring agricultural scientists, marketing professionals, and vermitechnology experts.
- Comprehensive deliberations on:
    - Forward and backward market linkages.
    - Value addition of raw produce.
    - Establishing buyback agreements with ISM&H pharmaceutical companies.

The session concluded with several actionable recommendations to strengthen the medicinal crop value chain through integrated institutional frameworks and policy support.

Conclusion

The well-orchestrated dissemination strategy—comprising institutional support, knowledge-sharing events, expert training, and continuous farmer engagement—played a transformative role in mainstreaming medicinal crop cultivation in Western Uttar Pradesh. What began as a pioneering initiative gradually evolved into a farmer-driven movement. Field surveys conducted during 2022–23 confirmed this impact, revealing marked improvements in farmer awareness, cultivation practices, and income levels from medicinal crop farming.

CHAPTER 7

ESTABLISHMENT OF DEMONSTRATION PLOTS ON MEDICINAL CROPS

Demonstration plots serve as practical learning sites for farmers, showcasing innovative agricultural techniques and enabling them to assess the economic viability of cultivating new crops. These "model farms" are typically small landholdings (ranging between 0.25 to 0.5 acres), owned and managed by selected progressive farmers under the continuous technical guidance of agricultural experts. These plots offer hands-on exposure to Good Agricultural Practices (GAP), including land preparation, input management, pest and disease control, and post-harvest handling.

Strategically located near roadways for maximum visibility, these demonstration plots act as knowledge hubs for neighboring farmers, offering them real-time insights into the practical aspects of medicinal crop cultivation.

7.1 Demonstration Plots at Farmers' Fields

During 2003–2004, a total of 35 demonstration plots were established across nine development blocks in Aligarh and Hathras districts. The initiative aimed to promote field-level awareness and hands-on training in the cultivation of high-demand medicinal crops such as Jatropha, Kaunch, Ashwagandha, Sanai, Mushkdana, and Kalmegh.

Demonstration Plots on Medicinal Crops

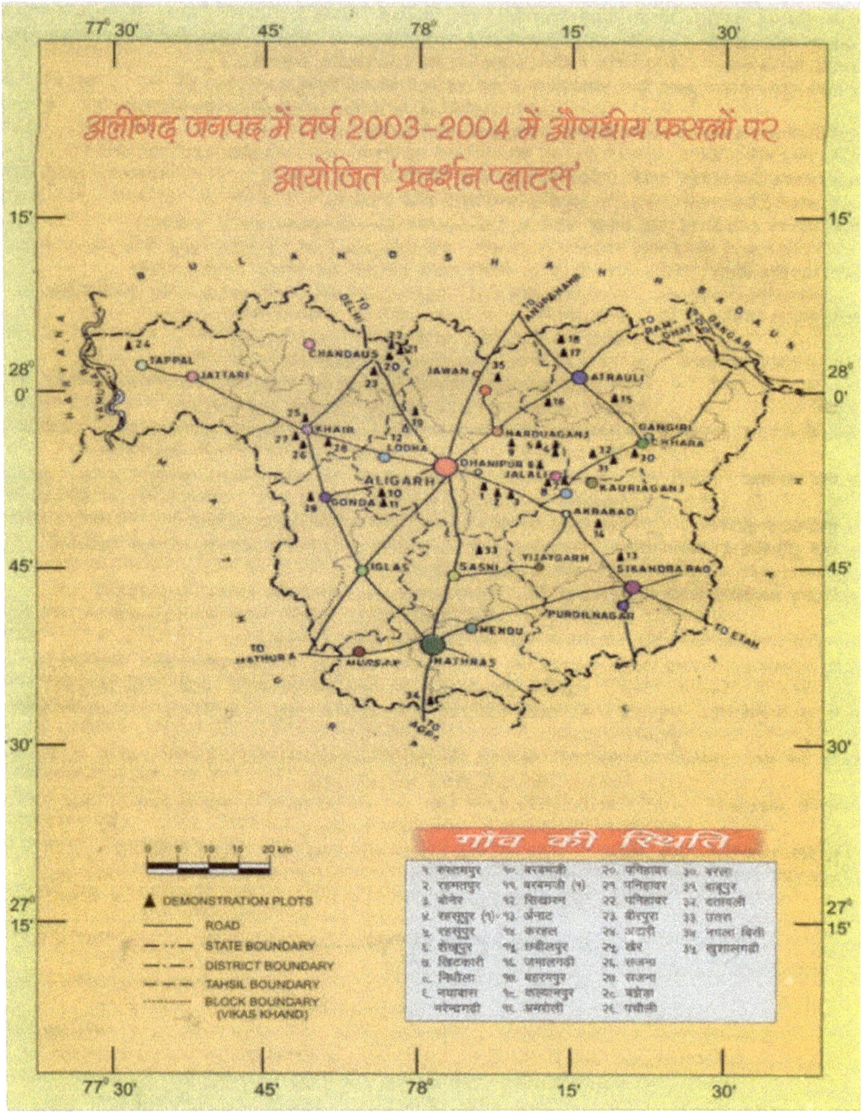

Fig 7.1: Mapping of 35 Medicinal Crops 'Demonstration Plots' Across Villages in District Aligarh (2003-2004)

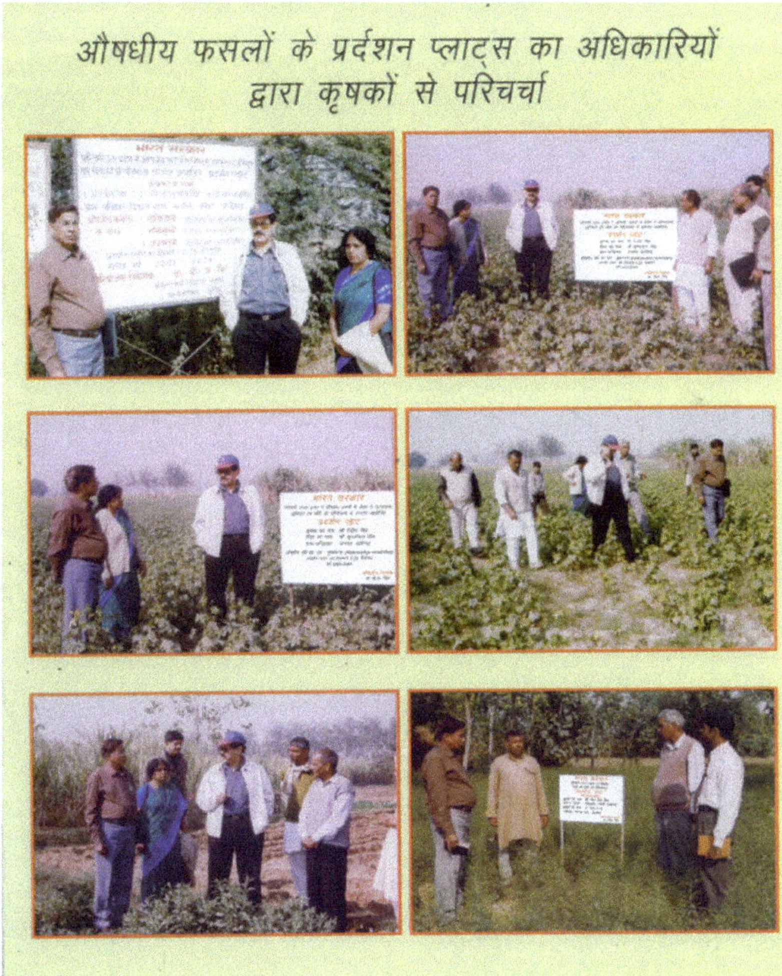
औषधीय फसलों के प्रर्दशन प्लाट्स का अधिकारियों
द्वारा कृषकों से परिचर्चा

Fig 7.2: Dr. R.B.S. Rawat, former CEO, National Medicinal Plants Board Engaging with Farmers and Reviewing Medicinal Crops Demonstration Plots in Village Panihavar, District Aligarh

Out of 110 farmers who expressed interest, 35 were selected as per project guidelines. These farmers received free quality planting material and continuous technical assistance from the project team. The demonstration plots provided the first-ever live experience for these farmers in cultivating medicinal crops under expert supervision.

The distribution of demonstration plots across blocks in Aligarh district is summarized below:

Table 7.1:

S. No.	Block Name	Medicinal Crops Cultivated	No. of Demonstration Plots
1	Dhanipur	Kalmegh, Ashwagandha, Sonamukhi	9
2	Lodha	Kalmegh, Sonamukhi	3
3	Gangiri	Kalmegh, Ashwagandha	4
4	Chandaus	Sonamukhi, Ashwagandha, Mushkdana	4
5	Jawan	Jatropha, Kalmegh, Sonamukhi	4
6	Khair	Kaunch, Ashwagandha	5
7	Gonda	Ashwagandha, Kalmegh	2
8	Sikandrarao	Ashwagandha, Mushkdana	2
9	Sasni	Kalmegh, Mushkdana	2
	Total		**35**

7.2 Organizing Farmers Field Day (FFD)

To consolidate the learning from these demonstration plots, a Farmers Field Day (FFD) was organized on 22nd November 2003 at Panihavar village, Gabhana, Aligarh district. The event served as a platform for farmers and researchers exchange insights and assess the impact of medicinal plant cultivation in Western Uttar Pradesh.

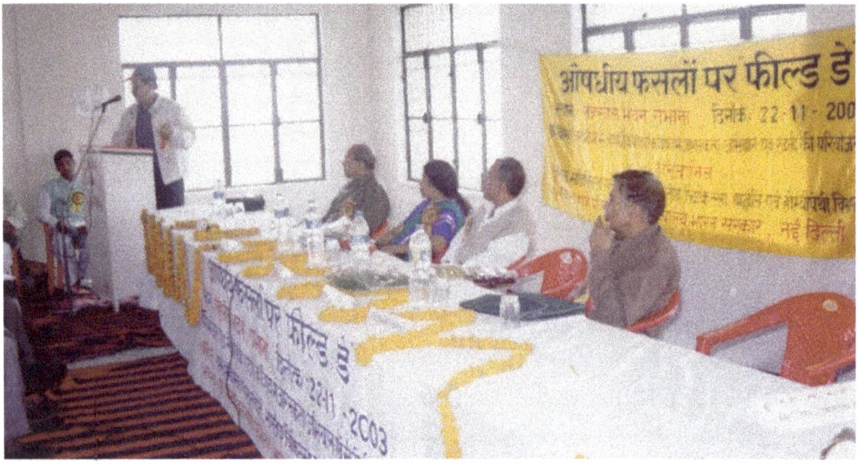

Fig 7.3 : Former CEO of National Medicinal Plants Board, New Delhi, Dr. RBS Rawat Speaks at Farmers' Meet at Gabhana, District Aligarh on Field Day Celebrations on 22nd November 2003

The Field Day was presided over by the Chief Executive Officer, National Medicinal Plants Board (NMPB), Government of India, and attended by over 202 farmers and stakeholders from districts including Etah, Agra, Aligarh, Mainpuri, and Hathras.

Key highlights of the event included:

- Sharing of field results by progressive farmers engaged in medicinal crop cultivation under the project.
- Interactive discussions on challenges and opportunities in the sector.
- Expert sessions on vermitechnology, crop-specific practices, and marketing strategies.
- Buy-back arrangements for the produce harvested from demonstration plots.

Farmers were repeatedly advised to:

- Follow the "Instructions Before Cultivation of Medicinal Plants" circulated under the project.
- Conduct cost-benefit analyses before expanding the area under cultivation.
- Ensure pre-arranged market linkages to safeguard against exploitation.
- Consider the formation of crop-specific farmer federations such as 'Mushkdana Federation' and 'Kalmegh Federation' to secure better prices and bargaining power.

Many farmers reported that they had already secured buyers for their produce from demonstration plots, indicating early market success. The Field Day reinforced confidence among farmers in adopting medicinal crop cultivation as a sustainable and profitable agricultural venture.

This systematic and participatory approach—combining demonstration plots with training events like the Farmers' Field Day—laid a robust foundation for scaling up medicinal plant farming in Western Uttar Pradesh.

CHAPTER 8

MODEL FARMING OF MEDICINAL CROPS — DEVELOPING MEDICINAL SEED VILLAGE

8.1 Concept of a Medicinal Seed Village

A *Medicinal Seed Village* is a designated rural cluster where a trained group of farmers actively engages in the production of high-quality seeds of medicinal crops. These farmers not only fulfill their own seed requirements but also supply to neighboring cultivators in a timely and cost-effective manner. The initiative is designed to upgrade the quality of farm-saved seeds and promote localized seed self-sufficiency.

To support this effort, financial assistance of 100% of the cost of foundation or certified seeds is provided, along with technical know-how for the cultivation of medicinal crops.

The objectives of the Medicinal Seed Village program include:

1. Selection of suitable villages through proposals received from respective Gram Sabhas.
2. Mobilization of farmers to collectively cultivate high-demand medicinal species with assured markets.
3. Provision of technical and material inputs including seeds, training, and crop management resources.
4. Facilitation of farmer federations for joint marketing and promotion of cooperative practices within the medicinal plant sector.

In essence, the programme aims:

- To train farmers in the production of quality seeds for medicinal crops and promote peer-to-peer seed availability.
- To ensure disease- and pest-free seed production through the use of appropriate plant protection measures.
- To promote seed production in compact and clustered areas.
- To achieve self-sufficiency and self-reliance at the village level in medicinal seed production.

8.2 Benefits of the Medicinal Seed Village

- Timely availability of seeds: Farmers have ready access to quality seeds at their doorstep during the appropriate sowing season.
- Trust and traceability: Farmers gain confidence in seed quality as the source is known and locally accessible.
- Accelerated adoption: New cultivars and varieties of medicinal crops can be disseminated more rapidly among farming communities.

8.3 Badagaon-Okhlana: The First Medicinal Seed Village in Uttar Pradesh

In alignment with this concept, Badagaon-Okhlana in Dhanipur Development Block, Aligarh district, Uttar Pradesh, was developed as a demonstration model of a Medicinal Seed Village under the ongoing project activities during 2005–06.

Process of Development:

During June–July 2005, project officials held several interactive sessions with farmers in the village. These meetings focused on:

- Awareness about commercially valuable medicinal crops.
- Training in scientific cultivation techniques.
- Cost-benefit analysis, post-harvest practices, and storage methods.
- Pest and disease management in medicinal crops.
- Market opportunities and long-term sustainability.

Following this outreach, 36 farmers (Appendix i) expressed willingness to participate in the initiative. They were provided free, quality planting materials for selected medicinal crops including:

- Ashwagandha *(Withania somnifera)*
- Kalmegh (*Andrographis paniculata)*
- Jatropha *(Jatropha curcas)*
- Kaunch *(Mucuna pruriens)*
- Sanai *(Cassia angustifolia)*
- Safed Musli *(Chlorophytum borivilianum)*
- Bael *(Aegle marmelos)*
- Amla *(Emblica officinalis)*

Cultivation was undertaken on approximately 32 acres of land under the technical supervision of project experts. (Details of farmers participating in this program with cultivation details are provided in Appendix I.)

Supplementary Initiatives:

To promote sustainable agricultural practices, a Vermicompost Unit was also established in the village. Furthermore, the participating farmers organized themselves into a federation to facilitate collective marketing, enabling them to secure remunerative prices and reduce dependency on middlemen and traders.

8.4 Strategic Significance and Recognition

The development of Badagaon-Okhlana as a *model Medicinal Seed Village* was the first of its kind in Uttar Pradesh and was aligned with national development goals for the medicinal plant sector.

Notably, the initiative resonated with the vision of former President of India, Dr. A.P.J. Abdul Kalam, who had advocated for the establishment of *Village Knowledge Centers*—to act as grassroots helpdesks, build local confidence, and serve as e-governance hubs to empower rural communities (Times of India, August 28, 2005).

This effort represented a proactive step toward supporting the Government of India's mission to boost the cultivation, processing, and marketing of medicinal plants, especially those in high demand by the Indian Systems of Medicine and Homeopathy (AYUSH).

8.5 Inauguration and Farmer Engagement

The formal inauguration of the *Badagaon-Okhlana Medicinal Seed Village* – first in the state, was held on 27th November 2005 and was graced by Shri B. S. Sajwan, then Chief Executive Officer, National Medicinal Plants Board (NMPB), Government of India.

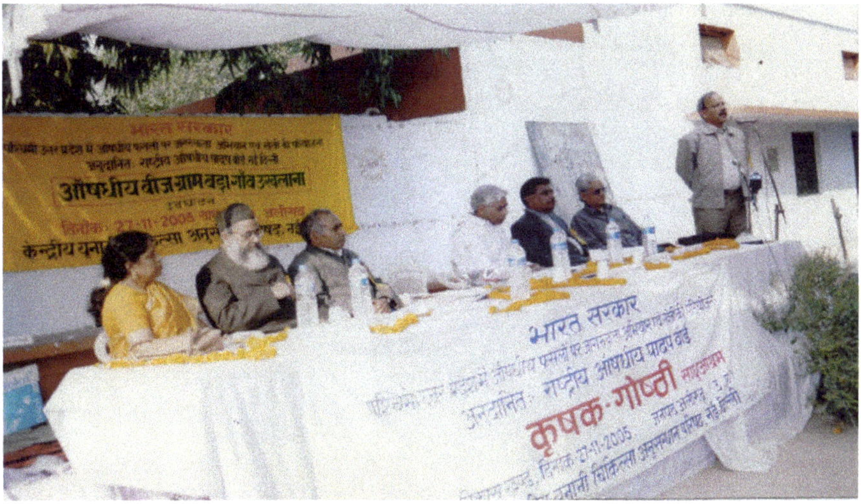

Fig 8.1: Mr. B.S. Sajwan, IFS, former CEO, National Medicinal Plants Board, New Delhi, Inaugurating the Medicinal Seed Village at Baragaon okhlana in district Aligarh and Addressing the Farmers on 27th November 2005

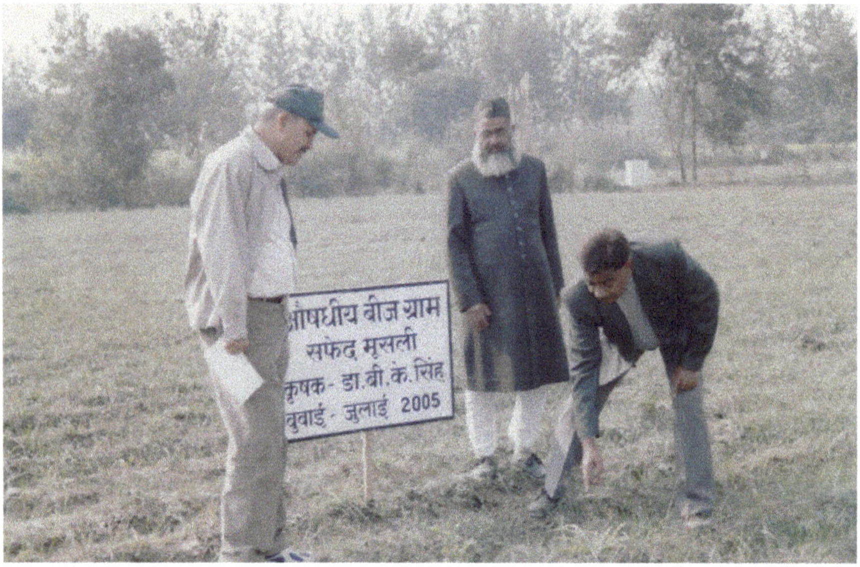
औषधीय बीज ग्राम
सफेद मूसली
कृषक - डा.बी.के.सिंह
बुवाई - जुलाई 2005

Fig 8.2: Mr. B.S. Sajwan, former CEO of National Medicinal Plants Board, New Delhi, Reviewing the Cultivation of 'Safed Musli' in Medicinal Seed Village Baragoan Okhlana in district Aligarh

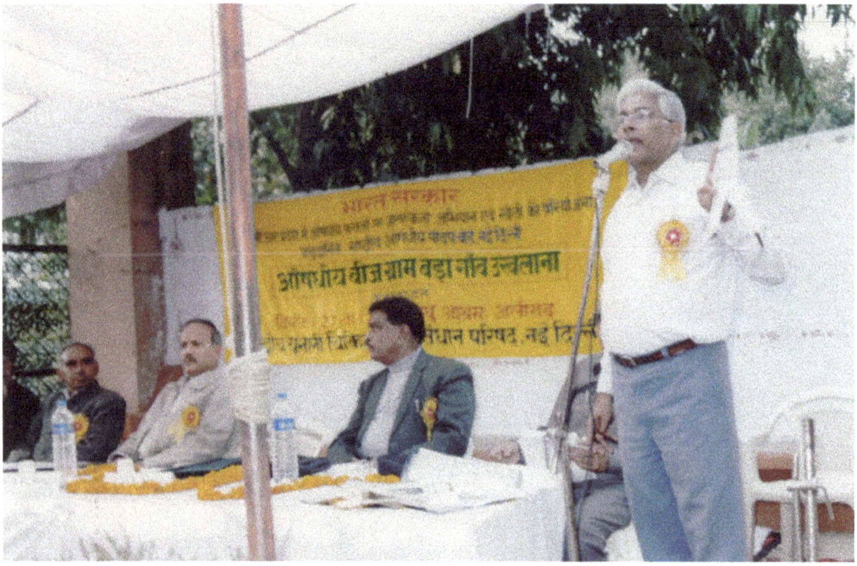

Fig 8.3 : Dr. V.K. Singh, Project Director, Addressing Farmers on the Occasion of Inauguration of Medicinal Seed Village at Baragaon Okhlana in district Aligarh on 27th November 2005

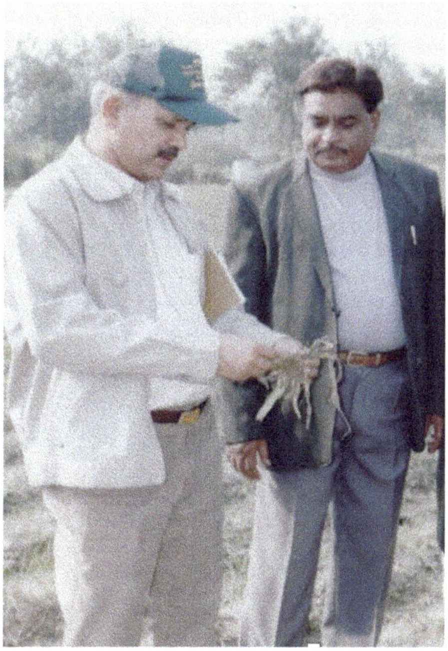

Fig 8.4 Mr. B.S. Sajwan, former CEO, National Medicinal Plants Board, New Delhi, Inspecting the crop of 'Safed Musli' on 27th November 2005 . Standing with him is Dr. B.K. Singh, Progressive Farmer Cultivating the Crop in Medicinal Seed Village, Baragaon Okhlana, District Aligarh

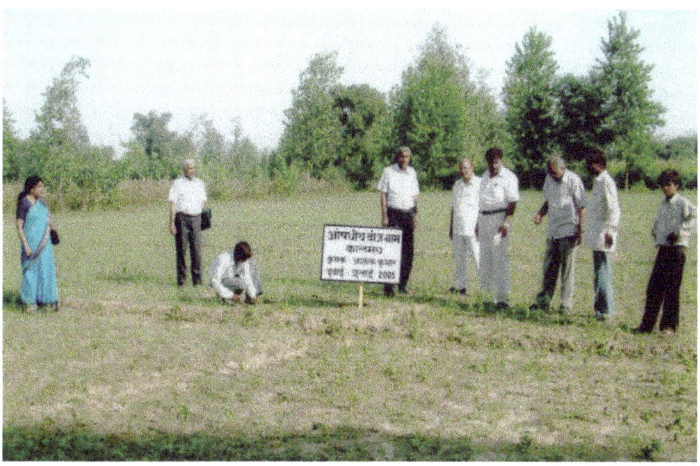

Fig 8.5 :A View of Inspection of Kalmegh (Andrographis paniculata) Medicinal Crop Field by Members of Project Steering Committee at Baragoan Okhlana, District Aligarh on 3rd October 2005

Shri Sajwan also addressed a gathering of 157 progressive medicinal plant farmers at Atrauli, where he commended the project's efforts in establishing this model seed village.

On this occasion, participating farmers were provided with a 'Sumangal Diary', a cultivation logbook designed to help them systematically record day-to-day field operations, monitor crop growth, and assess overall performance for continuous improvement.

Conclusion

The establishment of *Badagaon-Okhlana* as Uttar Pradesh's first Medicinal Seed Village marked a transformative step in the region's approach to medicinal plant cultivation. Through dedicated farmer training, technical support, input delivery, and cooperative marketing, the initiative laid the foundation for scalable, sustainable, and locally-managed medicinal seed systems. This model not only enhanced farmer incomes and self-reliance but also contributed to the national goal of expanding the medicinal plants sector through grassroots participation.

CHAPTER 9

ORGANIC FARMING BY FARMERS – SETTING UP OF A VERMICOMPOST UNIT

9.1 Introduction to Organic Farming in Medicinal Crop Cultivation

In recent years, organic farming has attracted growing attention from scientists, policymakers, and farmers alike due to its potential to create an integrated, humane, and ecologically sustainable agricultural system. This approach is especially relevant in the cultivation of medicinal and traditional plants, where ecological integrity and quality assurance are of paramount importance.

The overarching goal of organic farming in the medicinal plant sector is to produce high-quality raw materials that comply with pharmaceutical standards, while ensuring long-term soil fertility, biodiversity conservation, and sustainability of production systems.

A cornerstone of organic farming is the elimination of synthetic inputs, including chemical fertilizers, pesticides, and herbicides, which are prohibited under various organic certification frameworks in Europe, North America, and increasingly in India. Instead, organic farming relies on natural, farm-based inputs to nourish the soil, maintain ecological balance, and support the biological processes essential for the optimal therapeutic efficacy of medicinal plants.

9.2 Importance of Organic Inputs

Organic fertilizers play a vital role in this system. They supply essential nutrients gradually and improve soil structure and stability, thereby supporting the biosynthesis of active phytochemicals in medicinal crops. As such, organic farming contributes not only to soil conservation, fertility, and resilience but also to the economic viability of medicinal crop production by enhancing quality and marketability.

Recognizing the significance of organic farming in the Medicinal Seed Village Programme, a Vermicompost Unit was established in two villages of Aligarh district, Baragaon Okhlana and Panihavar, to serve as a demonstration model for the farmers. The aim was to empower local communities to produce their own organic compost, reduce dependency on chemical inputs, and promote sustainable cultivation of medicinal plants.

9.3 Vermicompost Unit Initiative

The initiative was launched to educate farmers on the methods and benefits of producing vermicompost through vermiculture and using it in organic agriculture—particularly in medicinal plant farming. In addition to promoting environmentally safe farming practices, this initiative also aimed to create self-employment opportunities in rural areas.

9.4 Technique of Vermicompost Preparation

Vermiculture refers to the practice of rearing earthworms—such as *Eisenia foetida*, *Perionyx excavatus*, and *Eudrilus eugeniae*—on degradable organic waste materials including kitchen waste, crop residues, and animal dung. In North India, *Eisenia foetida* (commonly known as red earthworms) are widely used for large-scale vermicomposting due to their efficiency.

The standard vermibed has dimensions of 10 feet × 3 feet × 1.5 feet and requires approximately 1 kg of earthworms to process around 5 quintals of organic waste. This waste is converted into nutrient-rich vermicompost within 45 to 50 days. Vermibeds can be constructed in open areas under shade trees or temporary huts, and should be regularly watered to maintain around 40% moisture.

To promote earthworm activity, vermibeds should be covered with 3–4 layers of agricultural waste mulch, which helps maintain darkness and consistent moisture levels.

9.5 Village Implementation: Baragaon Okhlana and Panihavar

Using the above technique, Vermicompost Units were successfully established in Baragaon Okhlana and Panihavar villages as part of the Medicinal Seed Village initiative. These units served as live demonstration models, enabling farmers to observe the process and outcomes firsthand.

Training sessions were conducted in the villages, during which farmers were guided through each step of vermicompost preparation—from selection of organic waste, setting up vermibeds, to monitoring compost maturation. The farmers were encouraged to use the produced vermicompost in their own medicinal crop fields, thereby improving soil health and reducing input costs without compromising on crop quality.

Farmers Training on Vermicompost Preparation

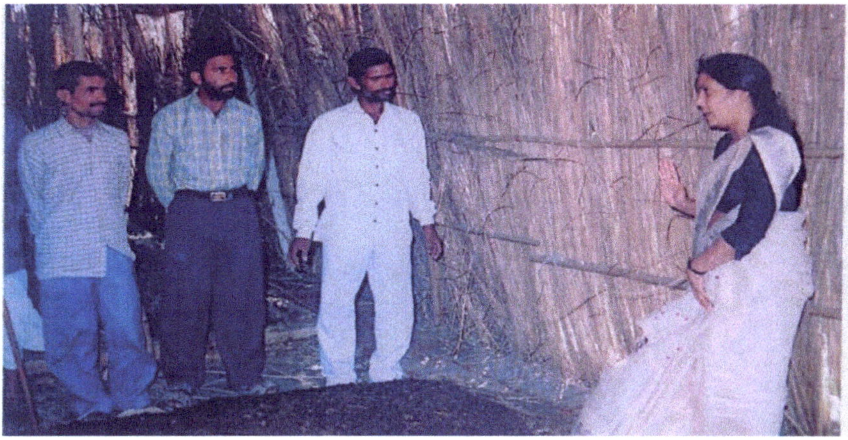

Fig 9.1 :Professor Shweta Yadav explaining the precautions to Farmers of Medicinal Seed Village, Baragaon Okhlana in District Aligarh in the preparation of Vermibeds and their proper upkeep until vermicompost is finally ready for use on 9th September 2005

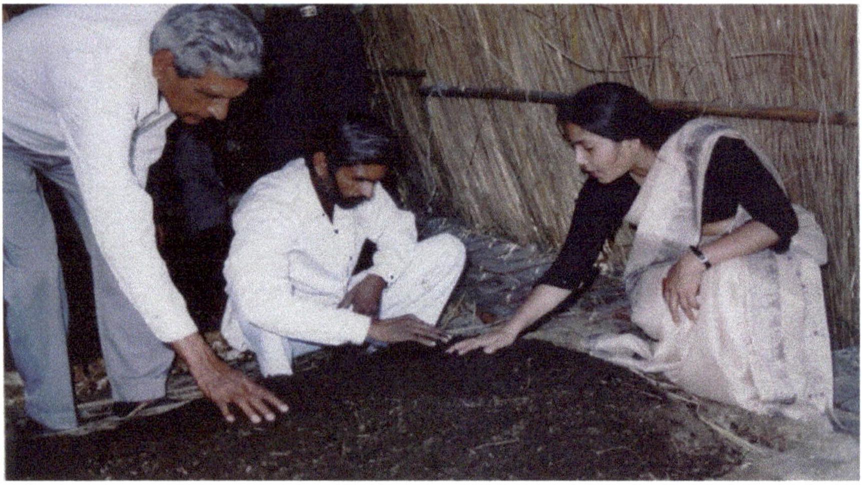

Fig 9.2: Professor Shweta Yadav, Assisted by Mr. R.P.P. Singh, Agriculture Officer (Project), Conducts Hands-on Vermicomposting Training for Farmers in Medicinal Seed Village at Baragoan Okhlana in district Aligarh on 9th September 2005.

By equipping rural farmers with knowledge and tools to produce cost-effective and eco-friendly organic inputs, this initiative has strengthened the foundation of sustainable medicinal plant farming in Western Uttar Pradesh. It stands as a replicable model for other regions aiming to integrate organic practices in herbal agriculture.

CHAPTER 10

MARKETING ASSISTANCE TO FARMERS FOR SELLING THEIR MEDICINAL PRODUCE

In order to support farmers in marketing their medicinal produce (crude drugs) and ensuring they receive fair and remunerative prices, a comprehensive and updated directory of buyers has been compiled. This directory includes manufacturers, suppliers, traders, exporters, and importers involved in the trade of raw materials used in Indian Systems of Medicine and Homeopathy (ISM&H).

Special emphasis has been placed on listing buyers located in nearby districts and states, to help reduce transportation costs for farmers and improve logistical efficiency. This initiative has been especially helpful for cultivators in rural and semi-urban parts of Western Uttar Pradesh and adjacent regions.

10.1 Compilation of the Buyer Directory

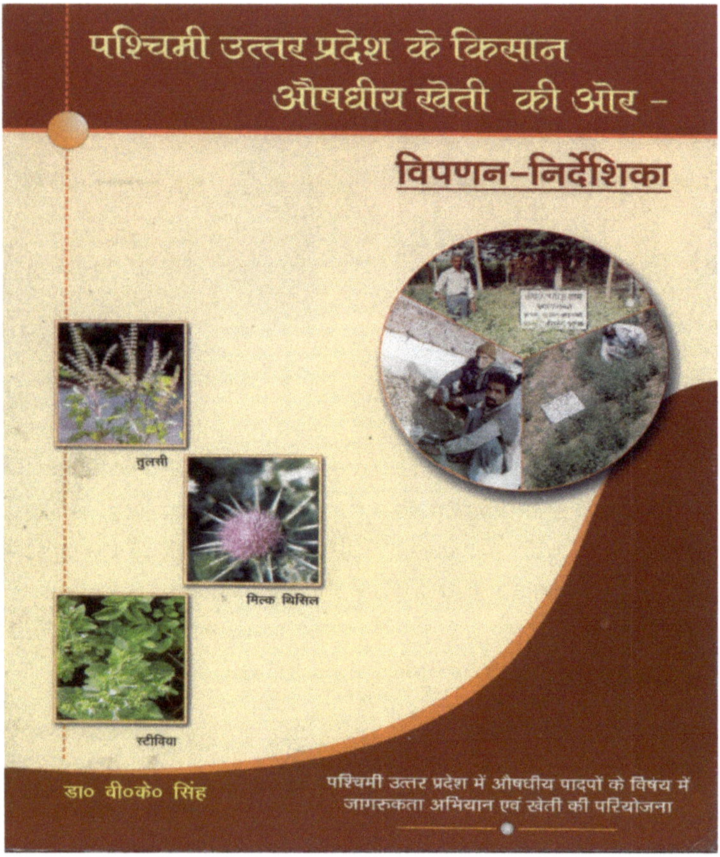

Fig 10.1: Medicinal Crops Market Opportunities: A Directory for Growers, Traders, and Buyers

As part of the project, a total of 2,279 addresses of buyers from Uttar Pradesh and Uttarakhand have been compiled and classified as follows:

1. Manufacturers of ISM&H pharmaceuticals – 1,059
2. Dealers, suppliers, and traders of raw drug materials – 146
3. Exporters of medicinal raw drugs – 56
4. Importers of medicinal raw drugs – 18

This directory serves as a practical marketing tool for farmers, enabling them to directly connect with reliable buyers and avoid exploitation by middlemen.

10.2 Capacity Building and Marketing Awareness

Since the beginning of project activities in 2002, participating farmers have progressively adopted the cultivation of medicinal plants in their fields. By 2006, many of these farmers had accumulated substantial experience in field production. At this juncture, it was deemed essential to equip them with advanced knowledge in marketing and quality maintenance of medicinal crops.

Accordingly, relevant information on best practices in marketing and post-harvest management has been included in the present guidebook. These topics are critical to help farmers understand the commercial value chain and improve both the marketability and shelf life of their produce.

Topics Covered in the Marketing Support Section

To strengthen farmers' knowledge and self-reliance in marketing, the following key areas have been addressed:

- **Good Agricultural Practices (GAP):**
  Guidelines to ensure the cultivation of medicinal plants meets quality and safety standards as per industry norms.

- **Good Storage Practices (GSP):**
  Methods for safe, hygienic, and contamination-free storage of harvested raw drugs to preserve their active ingredients and potency.

- **Supply Chain of Raw Medicinal Produce:**
  Insights into the pricing range between cultivators and end-users (processors, manufacturers) and how value is added along the chain.

- **Distribution Channels:**
  An overview of intermediaries, direct selling options, cooperative marketing, and contract farming models.

- **Major Marketing Centers in India:**
  A list of key wholesale and bulk markets for medicinal raw drugs in various states where farmers can access larger buyer networks.

- **Marketing Structure and Dynamics:**
  Understanding how the medicinal plant market functions, including price fluctuations, demand trends, and buyer preferences.

- **Quality Control Based on GAP:**
  Ensuring the produce adheres to quality benchmarks through compliance with Good Agricultural Practices, increasing both domestic and export viability.

- **Vermifarming Integration:**
  Promoting the use of **vermicompost** to improve crop quality organically, which aligns with the increasing demand for chemical-free herbal raw materials.

This chapter underlines the importance of farmer-market linkages, not just for financial benefit but for the long-term sustainability of the medicinal plant farming ecosystem. By equipping farmers with the necessary tools, contacts, and knowledge, this initiative bridges the gap between cultivation and commercialization, paving the way for a robust and farmer-friendly herbal market infrastructure.

CHAPTER 11

DELIVERABLES OF THE STUDY AND PROBLEMS FACED BY FARMERS IN MARKETING THEIR MEDICINAL PRODUCE

11.1 Overview of Activities and Key Deliverables

Over a span of three years (2002–2006), a range of impactful activities were undertaken as part of the medicinal crops cultivation and promotion initiative in Western Uttar Pradesh. These activities were designed to mobilize, educate, and empower farmers to transition into the cultivation of high-demand medicinal crops.

Key deliverables include:

- **Farmer Engagement & Knowledge Dissemination:**
  A total of 15 Farmers' Meets were organized across various development blocks—Dhanipur, Jawa, Gonda, Atrauli, Lodha, Hathras, Firozabad Narkhi, Awagarh, and Jalesar—covering the districts of Aligarh, Etah, Hathras, and Firozabad. Additionally, a National Seminar was held in Aligarh to bring together experts, practitioners, and farmers on a common platform.

- **Demonstration Plots:**
  Thirty-five demonstration plots were established in nine blocks—Dhanipur, Lodha, Gangiri, Chandaus, Jawa, Sasni, Gonda, Khair, and Sikandrabad—to showcase the cultivation practices of high-demand medicinal crops and encourage farmer participation.

- **Expansion of Cultivation:**
  As a result of these efforts, a total of 161.85 acres of farmland were brought under medicinal crop cultivation across different districts in the Agra Commissionary.

- **Provision of Quality Planting Material:**
  Farmers received a total of 203 kilograms of organically certified seeds, including Safed Musli, Isabgol, Sanai, Kalmegh, Mushkdana, Ashwagandha, Jatropha, Kaunch, Chandrashoor, and Kantakari, along with 90 Amla plants and 610 Bael plants.

Despite the substantial outreach and initial successes, the promotional activities remain largely unorganized. There is an urgent need for a structured and integrated approach to link cultivation with marketing, preferably by setting up district-level base centers.

11.2 Establishment of Model Seed Villages

Based on the rationale of creating integrated hubs, a "Medicinal Seed Village" was developed in Badagaon-Okhlana village (Dhanipur Block, Aligarh district). A group of 36 enthusiastic farmers were identified and supported to cultivate select high-demand medicinal plants with assured markets, along with the capacity to generate their own quality planting materials.

This model aims to:

- Ensure genuine and high-quality raw materials for manufacturers of ISM&H drugs.
- Improve the economic status of rural farmers by encouraging a shift from conventional crops to high-value medicinal crops.
- Promote sustainability through cultivation, reducing dependence on wild collection of medicinal plants.

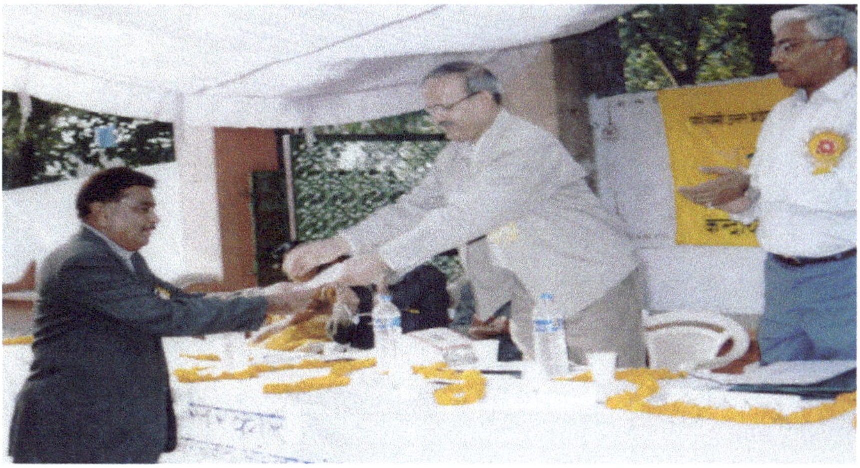

Fig 11.1 Farmer Empowerment in Action: Dr. B.K. Singh, A Professor of Chemistry and Progressive Farmer from Baragaon Okhlana, District Aligarh Receives Cheque from Mr. B.S. Sajwan, former CEO, National Medicine Plants Board for Safed Musli (Chlorophytom borivillanum) Produce, Sold Through Medicinal Crop Cultivation Project in Western U.P.

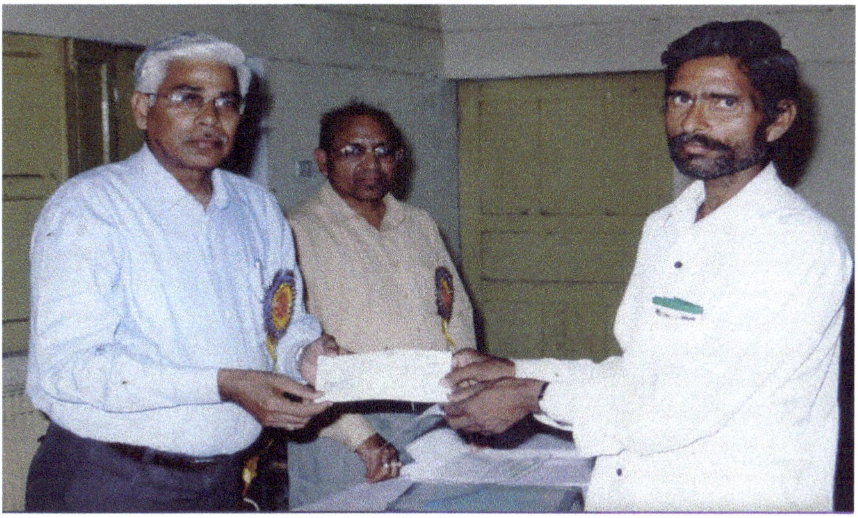

Fig 11.2 :Dr. V.K. Singh, Project Director (left) Presenting a Cheque to a Farmer (right) at Bijoli Development Block During a Farmers' Meet for his Produce of Ashwagandha Roots (Withania somnifera) Sold Through the Medicinal Crop Cultivation Project in Western U.P. .Dr. A.K. Tomar, Expert on Marketing, looks on.

Post-Harvest Processing of Medicinal Produce by Farmers

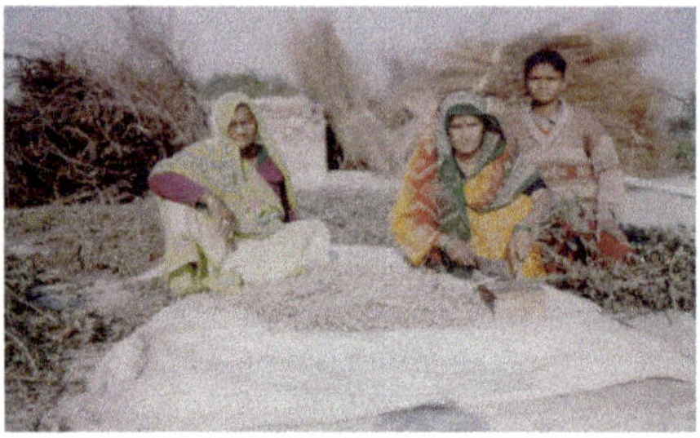

a

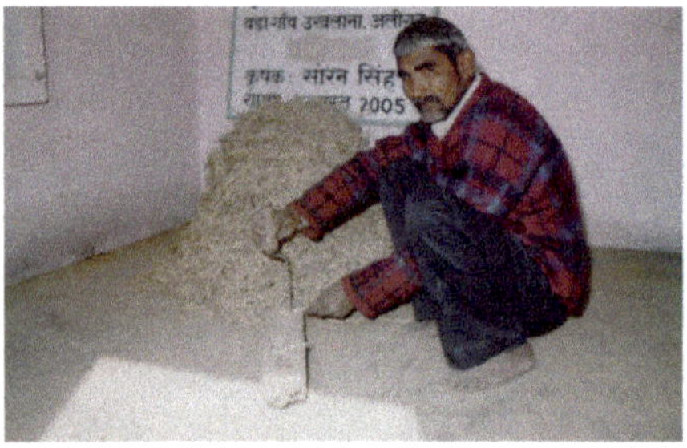

b

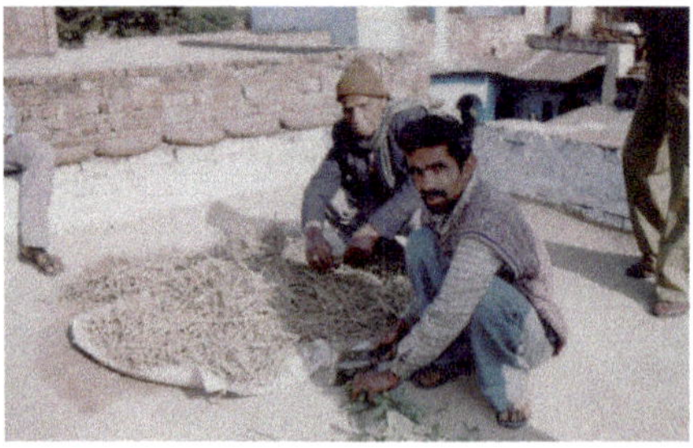

c

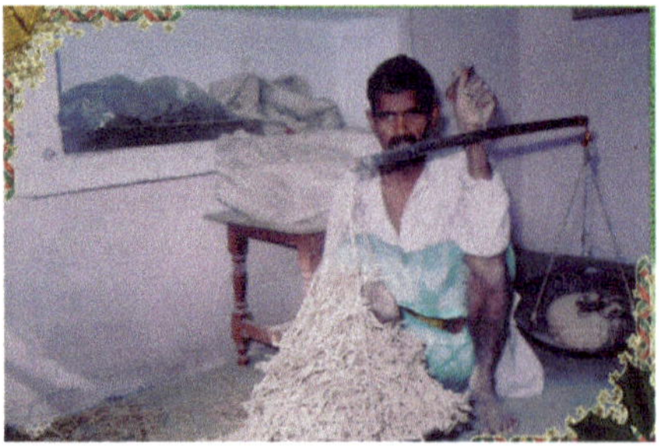

d

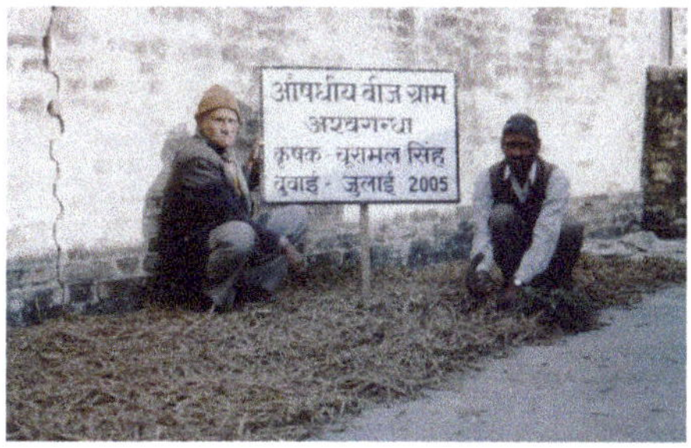
औषधीय बीज ग्राम
अश्वगन्धा
कृषक- चूरामल सिंह
बुवाई - जुलाई 2005

e

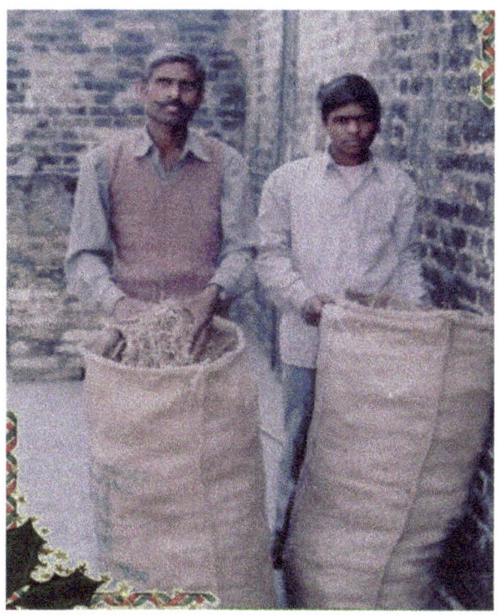

f

Fig 11.3 (a-f) Capturing the milestone: Joyous Farmers in Baragaon Okhlana process their first Ashwagandha (Withania somnifera) crop for market, in visuals.

11.3 Problems Faced by Farmers in Marketing Their Medicinal Produce

While the cultivation aspect of the project has been highly successful, a major challenge persists in the marketing of the harvested medicinal produce.

Key issues include:

- **Absence of Assured Marketing Channels:**
  Farmers often find themselves in a dilemma due to the lack of guaranteed procurement of their medicinal produce. Without

assured buy-back mechanisms, their income remains uncertain, discouraging sustained cultivation.

- Inaction from Institutional Bodies:
  Despite the establishment of the National Medicinal Plants Board (NMPB) under the Ministry of AYUSH in 2000–2001, the board has not adequately addressed the core issue of market linkage for poor farmers even after more than two decades.
- Positive Policy Response:
  On September 24, 2020, a significant step was taken when an MoU was signed between the National Medicinal Plants Board (NMPB), New Delhi, and the ISM pharmaceutical industry body, ensuring the purchase of farmers' medicinal produce. While this initiative is currently limited in scale, it signals a promising shift toward structured procurement.
- Proposed Policy Recommendations:
  It is recommended that the ISM drug industries body procure at least 25% of its raw material from cultivated sources, to:
  - Encourage large-scale cultivation.
  - Ensure economic viability for farmers.
  - Guarantee the availability of authentic, high-quality raw materials for ISM drug manufacturing.

This model of linking cultivation to marketing will not only strengthen the herbal raw drug supply chain but also ensure the economic empowerment of rural farmers. The shift from wild harvesting to sustainable farming will contribute significantly to the conservation and responsible use of medicinal biodiversity.

11.4 Appeal to the Authorities – Letter to the PMO India:

Acknowledging this gap, the author of this book personally wrote to the Prime Minister's Office (PMO–India) and concerned ministries on May 17, 2020, requesting intervention to support farmers cultivating medicinal crops (other than those supported by NMBP projects).

Nirmala Sitharaman Ministry of Finance, Government of India PMO India Ministry of AYUSH, Government of India National Medicinal Plants Board Shripad Naik NITI Aayog MYGov Corona Hub

Mrs Nirmala Sitharaman Ji
Hon'ble Finance Minister,
Government of India, New Delhi

Subject: Allocation of Rs 4000 crores for herbal farming in India… Stimulus package regd…

Respected Madam,

In reference to allocation of Rs 4000 crores by your Ministry as a special package for Herbal Farming in India, with a clear objective of Hon'ble PM, to improve the financial status of farmers of the country, I wish to submit the ground reality of the issue.

1. Our farmers are masters of cultivation practices and can grow any crop without any formal training by experts.
2. Government proposes to undertake Herbal Farming in some 10,000 hectares of land through farming communities throughout India.
3. Surely, there would be bumper medicinal crops and we will have tons of genuine raw material for manufacturing Ayurvedic and Unani medicines. One can imagine the hard labour and efforts that a poor farmer will make to produce the herbs at his field with solemn assurance of Government of India that this whole initiative is to improve his financial condition.
4. Madam, The ground reality is that there is no taker to the herbal produce (raw drugs) of poor farmers and he will be no where to sell their produce in market. Consequently, farmers will be forced to sell their produce at throwaway prices or perish the grown up crop in the absence of any buy back mechanism in place. They will become more poor and curse the government.
5. Therefore, unless the government assures the farmers to purchase their produce through a buyback mechanism OR its made mandatory for Ayurvedic and Unani medicines manufacturers in

India to purchase raw materials from farmers, the efforts of government including pumping of Rs 4000crores in this ambitious program, very close to our PM's heart will be a total waste of money and will be justified on papers only. At the end of day farmers will be many times poorer than becoming rich. THIS IS GROUND REALITY.

6. As of now 99% of manufacturers of Ayurvedic and Unani medicines in India are purchasing raw drugs locally (for instance: Khari baoli in Delhi, housing 250+ raw drugs shops). The raw drugs materials available on these shops are never identified and of very poor quality, adulterated, many years old, stored in damp unhygienic conditions with no expiry date, often ingested with worms etc. However, prices of this raw material are very very cheap. This is the main reason why Ayurvedic and Unani medicines manufactures throughout India purchase substandard and spurious raw materials EARNING MAXIMUM PROFIT at the cost of human health.
7. The National Medicinal Plants Board (Ministry of AYUSH,Government of India), New Delhi, established way back in 2001, has miserably failed to address this issue and to evolve buyback mechanism for common farmers (not those farmers who have been sanctioned projects by NMPB) and not been able to solve this problem as yet. The common farmers in India can never benefit from cultivation of medicinal crops unless there is buyback mechanism in force between manufacturers of AYUSH medicines and farmers or Government ensures purchase of total raw materials produce. Of course, only those smart farmers who were able to get a project from the National Medicinal Plants Board, managed submitting buyback agreements from traders. And not the common farmers.

Request:

Madam, Government of India should think twice before pumping a huge funds of Rs 4000crores for herbal farming in India .

I may retriate, unless government of India ensures a mechanism of buyback of herbal produce of farmers OR It's made mandatory for manufacturers of AYUSH medicines in India to purchase raw materials from farmers only, I'm afraid, farmers will never, ever benefit in India. And entire money of Rs 4000crores pumped for this novel cause to uplift farmers economy will be a sheer waste and a futile exercise.

I shall be very grateful, madam, for your personal attention in the matter. With profound regards, sincerely,

Dr V.K. Singh Retd. Dy. Director
(Botany)/ScientistIV, CCRUM,
Ministry of AYUSH

11. 5 AYUSH Ministry inks MoU with Industry Bodies to promote Medicinal Plants cultivation

Posted On: 24 SEP 2020 7:03PM by PIB Delhi

In a historic event today, the National Medicinal Plants Board (NMPB), Ministry of AYUSH signed an MoU through virtual meeting with the major AYUSH and Herbal industry bodies covering a set of measures to promote medicinal plant cultivation.

The industry bodies which signed the MoU include ADMA (Ayurvedic Drug Manufacturer's Association), Mumbai; AMAM (Association for Manufactures of Ayurvedic Medicines), New Delhi; AMMOI Ayurvedic Medicines Manufacturers Organization of India), Thrissur; AHNMI (Association for Herbal and Nutraceutical Manufacturers of India), Mumbai; FICCI (Federation of Indian Industries), New Delhi and CII (Confederation of Indian Industry), New Delhi.

The signing ceremony was graced by the presence of Vd. Rajesh Kotecha, Secretary AYUSH who assured that his ministry would provide necessary support to resolve the issues related to the industry provided they form a combined team and approach with solutions to the respective problems faced by them. He further assured that the present govt is committed to the development of AYUSH systems.

The industry assured the NMPB that they will provide the buy-back guarantee to the farmers / gatherers on the NMPB supported medicinal plant cultivation and collection programs. Dr JLN Sastry, CEO, NMPB signed the MoU on behalf of Ministry of AYUSH while Mr. Chandrakant Bhanushali (ADMA), Mr. Pradeep Multani (AMAM), Dr Ramanathan (AMMOI), Mr. Sanjay Mariwala (AHNMI), Mr. Praveen Mittal (FICCI), Mr. Rajeev Vasudevan (CII) have represented respective bodies. Industry representatives agreed that this unique gesture of Ministry of AYUSH would provide the sustainable supply of quality raw material to AYUSH, Nutraceutical and Herbal industry.

MV/SK

(Release ID: 1658765)

11.6 Medicinal Crops Sector Development: Insights for Government Action:

1. *Establish a regulatory framework:* Develop policies and guidelines for the cultivation, procurement, and marketing of medicinal crops.
2. *Create a centralized platform:* Set up a national-level platform for farmers to sell their medicinal crops, ensuring transparency and fair pricing.
3. *Contract farming:* Encourage contract farming practices, where farmers can enter into agreements with pharmaceutical companies or authorized buyers, ensuring a stable market and prices.
4. *Support cooperative societies:* Promote the formation of farmer cooperatives or societies to collectively market and sell medicinal crops, enhancing bargaining power and reducing exploitation.
5. *Develop grading and quality standards:* Establish standardized quality control measures to ensure consistency and quality of medicinal crops, facilitating better pricing and market access.
6. *Provide training and capacity building:* Offer training programs for farmers on sustainable cultivation practices, quality control, and market trends.
7. *Create a database:* Develop a database of medicinal crop farmers, buyers, and market trends to facilitate informed decision-making.
8. *Financial support:* Offer subsidies, loans, or other financial incentives to farmers and small-scale entrepreneurs in the medicinal crop sector.

9. *Market research and development:* Conduct market research to identify new opportunities and trends, and support the development of value-added products.
10. *Public-private partnerships:* Foster partnerships between government agencies, private companies, and farmers to promote the medicinal crop sector.

11.7 Key Medicinal Crops Recommended to Farmers of Western U.P. for Cultivation.

S. No.	Common Name	Botanical Name
1	Amla	*Emblica officinalis* Gaertn
2	Ashwagandha	*Withania somnifera (L.) Dunal*
3	Bael	*Aegle marmelos* (L.) Corr.
4	Isabgol	*Plantago ovata* Forsk
5	Kalmegh	*Andrographis paniculata* Nees
6	Safed Musli	*Chlorophytum (borivillianum)* Sant.
7	Senna	*Cassia angustifolia* Vahl.
8	Shatavari	*Asparagus racemosus* Willd.
9	Tulsi	*Ocimum sanctum* Linn.
10	Kanta Karanj	*Caesalpinia bonducella* (L.) Flemming
11	Kasni	*Cichorium intybus* Linn.

11.8 Project - generated Publications: Pictorial Representation of Project Activities

*Singh, V.K. (2007): Cultivation of Medicinal Crops in Western U.P.—Awareness and Training to Farmers. Presented at the International Symposium of Medicinal and Aromatic Plants, Fort valley State University, Georgia, USA (March 19–23, 2007).

*Singh, V.K. (2023): Online lecture "Cultivation of Medicinal Crops: Enhancing Indian Farmers Livelihoods" delivered at the National Conclave "Doubling the Income of Farmers in India" organised by the International Goodwill Society of India (IGSI), Aligarh chapter (May 12, 2023).

CHAPTER 12

CULTIVATION OF MEDICINAL PLANTS IN INDIA: FROM PLANNING TO POST-HARVEST

This chapter serves as a practical guide for beginners interested in cultivating medicinal plants, focusing on important considerations before, during, and after cultivation. It incorporates economic insights, shelf-life data, and species-specific recommendations based on authentic Indian government sources and agricultural studies.

12.1 Key Precautions Before Starting Medicinal Plant Cultivation

Before initiating the cultivation of medicinal crops, it is essential to gather complete information about agronomic techniques, expected yields, market demand, and input/output economics. Aspiring cultivators should consult the following resources:

- *"Cultivation Practices of Some Commercially Important Medicinal Plants" (2002)* by the National Medicinal Plants Board (NMPB), Ministry of AYUSH.
- *"Agrotechniques and Economics of Some Important Medicinal Plants of India" (2004)* published by NMPB.

These references provide comprehensive data on propagation techniques, soil suitability, irrigation practices, pest management, and economic viability.

12.2 Medicinal Plants Recommended for Cultivation in India

India's diverse agro-climatic zones support the cultivation of a wide variety of medicinal herbs. The following tables summarize species with strong domestic and export potential.

Table 12.2 – Selected Medicinal Herbs Suitable for Cultivation Across India

S.No	Botanical Name	Part Used & Price (approx. 2024–25)	Market Demand
1	*Aloe vera*	Leaves: ₹400–500/q; Powder: ₹5–6 lakh/q	Very High (Domestic + Export)
2	*Artemisia annua*	Whole plant, especially aerial parts	High (Export – anti-malarial use)
3	*Asparagus racemosus* (Shatavari)	Roots: ₹6,000–8,000/q	High (Pharma, Ayurveda)
4	*Bacopa monnieri* (Brahmi)	Whole plant: ₹2,000–3,000/q	High
5	*Boerhaavia diffusa* (Punarnava)	Roots & Leaves: ₹1,500/q	High
6	*Cassia angustifolia* (Senna)	Leaves & Pods: ₹45,000–50,000/ton	Very High
7	*Catharanthus roseus* (Sadabahar)	Roots: ₹2,500/q; Leaves: ₹3,500/q	High (Pharma use – vincristine)
8	*Centella asiatica* (Gotu Kola)	Whole plant: ₹2,000–2,200/q	High
9	*Chlorophytum borivilianum* (Safed Musli)	Roots: ₹80,000–1,00,000/q	Very High
10	*Coleus forskohlii*	Roots: ₹4,000–5,000/q	High (Export)
11	*Evolvulus alsinoides* / *Convolvulus pluricaulis*	Whole plant: ₹2,000–2,500/q	Moderate to High
12	*Gloriosa superba*	Seeds: ₹15,000–20,000/q	High (Colchicine source)
13	*Glycyrrhiza glabra* (Mulethi)	Roots: ₹7,000–9,000/q	Very High
14	*Gymnema sylvestre* (Gudmar)	Leaves: ₹3,000–4,000/q	High (Anti-diabetic market)

S.No	Botanical Name	Part Used & Price (approx. 2024–25)	Market Demand
15	*Mentha spp.*	Menthol: ₹25,000/q	Very High
16	*Mucuna pruriens* (Kapikachhu)	Seeds: ₹5,000–6,000/q	High (L-Dopa source)
17	*Phyllanthus amarus / P. niruri*	Whole plant: ₹2,500–3,000/q	High
18	*Plantago ovata* (Isabgol)	Seeds: ₹4,500–5,500/q	Very High
19	*Rauwolfia serpentina* (Sarpgandha)	Roots: ₹8,000–10,000/q	High
20	*Solanum khasianum / S. indicum*	Fruits: ₹1,500/q	Moderate to High
21	*Tinospora cordifolia* (Guduchi)	Stem, Leaves: ₹2,000–2,500/q	Very High
22	*Tylophora indica* (Asthmatic root)	Roots: ₹4,000–6,000/q	Moderate
23	*Withania somnifera* (Ashwagandha)	Roots: ₹10,000–30,000/q	Very High

12.3 Government-Recommended Species for Large-Scale Cultivation

The Planning Commission's Task Force on Medicinal Plants recommends the following 25 species for sustainable cultivation due to their high therapeutic value and market potential:

Table 12.3 – Medicinal Plants Recommended for Cultivation by Task Force

S.No	Common Name	Botanical Name
1	Amla	*Emblica officinalis*
2	Ashwagandha	*Withania somnifera*
3	Ashoka	*Saraca asoca*
4	Atis	*Aconitum heterophyllum*
5	Baiberang	*Embelia ribes*
6	Bael	*Aegle marmelos*
7	Brahmi	*Bacopa monnieri*
8	Chandan	*Santalum album*
9	Chirata	*Swertia chirata*

S.No	Common Name	Botanical Name
10	Giloy	*Tinospora cordifolia*
11	Guggal	*Commiphora wightii*
12	Rasaut	*Berberis aristata*
13	Isabgol	*Plantago ovata*
14	Jatamansi	*Nardostachys jatamansi*
15	Kalmegh	*Andrographis paniculata*
16	Katuki	*Picrorhiza kurroa*
17	Kokum	*Garcinia indica*
18	Kuth	*Saussurea lappa*
19	Mulethi	*Glycyrrhiza glabra*
20	Pippali	*Piper longum*
21	Gudmar	*Gymnema sylvestre*
22	Shatavari	*Asparagus racemosus*
23	Shankhapushpi	*Convolvulus pluricaulis*
24	Safed Musli	*Chlorophytum borivilianum*
25	Senna	*Cassia angustifolia*

Table 12.4 – Shelf Life of Selected Medicinal Plants (as per Good Storage Practices - GSP)

S.No	Common Name	Botanical Name	Plant Part	Shelf Life
1	Amla	*Emblica officinalis*	Fruit, Leaf	1 year
2	Ashoka	*Saraca asoca*	Bark, Flower	2 years
3	Ashwagandha	*Withania somnifera*	Root, Leaf	1.5 years
4	Bael	*Aegle marmelos*	Fruit, Bark	2 years
5	Bhumi Amla	*Phyllanthus amarus*	Whole Plant	1 year
6	Brahmi	*Bacopa monnieri*	Whole Plant	1 year
7	Guduchi	*Tinospora cordifolia*	Stem	6 months
8	Gudmar	*Gymnema sylvestre*	Leaf	1.5 years
9	Isabgol	*Plantago ovata*	Husk	2 years
10	Kalihari	*Gloriosa superba*	Rhizome	2 years
11	Kalmegh	*Andrographis paniculata*	Whole Plant	1 year
12	Makoy	*Solanum nigrum*	Whole Plant	1 year
13	Mulethi	*Glycyrrhiza glabra*	Root	2 years
14	Safed Musli	*Chlorophytum borivilianum*	Root	2 years

S.No	Common Name	Botanical Name	Plant Part	Shelf Life
15	Sarpgandha	*Rauwolfia serpentina*	Root	2 years
16	Senna	*Cassia angustifolia*	Leaf, Pod	1.5 years
17	Shatavari	*Asparagus racemosus*	Root	1.5 years
18	Tulsi	*Ocimum sanctum*	Whole Plant	1 year

12.4 Economics of Medicinal Plants Cultivation (Per Acre Estimates)

Medicinal plant farming is a viable agri-business opportunity. Below are average input-output economics based on government and institutional data (NMPB, NABARD, ICAR, CSIR):

Table 12.5 – Cultivation Economics of Key Medicinal Plants (Per Acre – 2024)

S.No	Plant	Duration (Years)	Cost of Cultivation (₹)	Revenue (₹)	Expected Yield
1	Amla	6+	20,000	60,000+ annually	8–10 tons fruit
2	Ashoka	10	6,000	25,000+	Bark
3	Ashwagandha	1	7,000	22,000+	3 q dry root
4	Brahmi	1	18,000	55,000	20–25 q herbage
5	Giloy	1	3,000	7,500	4 q dry stem
6	Gudmar	4	3,500	8,000	4–5 q leaves
7	Isabgol	1	12,000	25,000	6 q seed
8	Kalihari	5	1,20,000	6,00,000	13 q seed or 30 q tuber
9	Kalmegh	1	9,000	14,000	12 q herbage
10	Kapikachhu	1	4,500	10,000	5 q seed
11	Makoy	1	6,000	20,000	5 q herbage
12	Mulethi	3	40,000	2,00,000+	30 q root
13	Muskdana	1	3,500	10,000	200 kg seed
14	Sadabahar	1	3,000	9,000	5 q herbage
15	Safed Musli	1	2,50,000	4,50,000	3.5 q dry root
16	Sarpgandha	2	25,000	50,000	6 q root
17	Senna	1	4,000	7,000	4 q dry leaf
18	Semal Musli	2	8,000	25,000	1 q root

S.No	Plant	Duration (Years)	Cost of Cultivation (₹)	Revenue (₹)	Expected Yield
19	Shatavari	2	25,000	60,000	35 q root
20	Stevia	1	2,00,000+	Market dependent	4–5 harvests
21	Tulsi	1	2,000	6,000+	20–25 kg oil

Note: Prices vary based on quality, location, and market linkages. Subsidies under the National AYUSH Mission and State Medicinal Plant Boards can significantly reduce input costs.

12.5 Policy Support and Subsidies in India (Updated 2024)

- The **National Medicinal Plants Board (NMPB)** under the Ministry of AYUSH offers financial assistance for cultivation through the **Medicinal Plants component of the National AYUSH Mission (NAM)**.
- Farmers can get up to **50–75% subsidy** on nursery establishment, cultivation, and post-harvest infrastructure depending on species and state-specific schemes.
- **State Medicinal Plant Boards (SMPBs)** in states like Madhya Pradesh, Chhattisgarh, and Uttarakhand are highly active in supporting growers.
- Tie-ups with **AYUSH clusters, herbal product manufacturers, and FPOs** (Farmer Producer Organizations) improve access to markets.

12.6 Conclusion

With India's growing herbal medicine sector—projected to reach USD 24 billion by 2026—medicinal plant cultivation is emerging as a high-potential green enterprise. Success depends on choosing the right species, using quality planting material, following GAP and GSP, and engaging with market players from the start. Government schemes and institutional support further enhance the viability of this venture for Indian farmers.

FURTHER READING

1. Anonymous (2000). Report of the Task Force on Conservation and Sustainable Use of Medicinal Plants. Planning Commission, Government of India, New Delhi.
2. Anonymous (2001). Herbal Products-Current Status, Vision and Action Plan. Report of the Scientific Advisory Committee to the Cabinet (SAC-C), Government of India, New Delhi. (Brought out by: TIFAC, New Delhi).
3. Anonymous (2002). Cultivation Practices of Some Commercially Important Medicinal Plants. National Medicinal Plants Board, Government of India, New Delhi.
4. Anonymous (2004) Agrotechniques and Economics of Some Important Medicinal Plants of India. NMPB, New Delhi, 2004.
5. Anonymous (2008). Agro-techniques of Selected Medicinal Plants, Vol.1. National Medicinal Plants Board, Government of India, New Delhi.
6. Anonymous (2014). Agrotechniques of selected Medicinal Plants, Vol. 2, National Medicinal Plants Board, Ministry of Ayush, Government of India, New Delhi 110001.
7. Anonymous (2002). Demand study for selected medicinal plants. Centre for Research, Planning and Action. Department of Indian Systems of Medicine and Homeopathy (ISM & H) & World Health Organisation (WHO)
8. Dadhich, Mahesh Kumar ; Sanwal, Chandra Shekhar ; Mahajan Bidhan ; Vaishya Jeetendre kumar ; Dutt Sunil, Rath Chinway ; Sharma Saurabh ; Tyagi Kavita ; Dwivedi, Himanshu ; Shukla, Chandra Prakash ; Murjeswaran R ; Sharma, Rajeev Kumar (2024).

Contribution of the National Medicinal Plants Board (NMPB), Ministry of AYUSH in the Medicinal Plant Sector – An appraisal. *International Journal of Ayurveda Research* 5(2): 62-75.

9. Ganesan A., Marichamy, K., Tnagamariappan (2016). Development of Medicinal Plants Sector in India-An Empirical Study. *Int. J. of Engineering Technology, Management and Applied Sciences*, 4, (1), 82-88.
10. Goswami, R., Chatterjee, S., Prasad B. (2014). Farm Types and Their Economic Characterization in complex Agro-Ecosystems for Informed Extension Intervention: Study from Coastal West Bengal, India. *Agric. Food Econ.*, 2: 1-14.
11. Invest India (Government of India) : One of the Fastest Growing Sectors in India
12. Joshi K ., Chavan P., Warnde D., Patwardhan B. (2004). Molecular Markers in Herbal Drug Technology. *Current Science*, 87 ; 159-167
13. Kala, C.P., Dhyani, P.P. and Sajwan, B.S. (2006). Review: Developing the medicinal plants sector in northern India: Challenges and opportunities. *Journal of Ethnobiology and Ethnomedicine* 2: 32. Doi 10.1186/1746-4269-2-32
14. Karki, Madhav and Rawat R.B.S., Uniyal, R. (2004). Revitalizing South Asian Heritage of Traditional Medicine & Medicinal Plants. Medicinal & Aromatic Plants Programme in Asia (MAPPA) & National Medicinal Plants Board, Department of Ayush, Ministry of Health and Family Welfare, Government of India, New Delhi.
15. Marshall, E. (2011). Health and Wealth from Medicinal and Aromatic Plants. Diversification Booklet No. 17. Rural Infrastructure and Agro-Industries Division, FAO: Rome, Italy.
16. Rathore R, Mathur A. (2018). Entrepreneurship Development in Medicinal and Aromatic Plants: Prospects and Challenge. *Int. J. Econ. Plants*, 5 32.35.
17. Rizvi Mohammad Afzal, Saeed Aftab, Zubairy Naimuddin (2007). Medicinal Plants-History, Cultivation and Uses. Hamdard Institute of Advanced Studies & Research, Karachi, Pakistan.

18. Samal, J. (2016). Medicinal Plants and related developments in India: A peep into 5-year plans of India. *Indian J. of Health Sciences*, 9 (1): 14-19.
19. Shakya, A.K. (2016). Medicinal Plants: Future Source of New Drugs. *Int. Herb. Med.*, 4, 59-64.
20. Singh, V.K. and Shamima Hashmi (2003). Pashchmi Uttar Pradesh me Aushdhiya Faslo ki Kheti (Sambhavna aur Vikas). National Medicinal Plants Board project, Government of India, New Delhi (In Hindi).
21. Singh, V.K. and Shamima Hashmi (2006). Pashchmi Uttar Pradesh me Aushdhiya Faslo ki Kheti (Sambhavna aur Vikas). National Medicinal Plants Board project, Government of India, New Delhi (Revised edition).
22. Singh, V.K. (2006). *Pashchmi Uttar Pradesh ke Kesan Aushdhiya Kheti ki Ore – Vipran Nirdeshika* (Marketing Directory for Medicinal Produce). National Medicinal Plants Board project, Government of India, New Delhi (In Hindi).
23. Singh, V.K. (2014, November 27-28). Conserving Bio-Diversity of High-Demand Medicinal Plants Through Ex-Situ Cultivation in Western Uttar Pradesh. Abstract retrieved *International Journal of Pharmacognosy.* (GL-16): 115. Proceedings of the Conference, "Modern Methods of Studies in Unani Medicine" (Eds A.Latif, Sumbul Rehman and others). Faculty of Unani Medicine, Aligarh Muslim University, Aligarh, India.
24. Ved, D.K. and Goraya, G.S. (2007). Demand and Supply of Medicinal Plants in India. National Medicinal Plants Board, New Delhi, & Foundation for Revitalisation of Local Health Traditions, Bangalore.

APPENDIX I

LIST OF PARTICIPATING FARMERS IN MEDICINAL SEED VILLAGE PROGRAM, BARAGOAN – OKHLANA (2005-2006), WITH CULTIVATION DETAILS.

List of Cultivators of Medicinal Seed Village Baragaon (Ukhalana), (Aligarh) With details of Kharif Crops Year 2005

SNO	Name of Farmer with Father's Name and Address	Ashwagandha(*Withania somnifera*),			Kalmegh(*Andrographis paniculata*)			Kaunch (*Mucuna pruriens*)			Bael Tree (*Aegle marmelos*)			Amla Tree (*Emblica officinalis*)			Kanta Karanj (*Caesalpinia bonduc* (L.) Roxb.			Jatropha (*Jatropha curcas*)		
		Seed Qty. in Kg	Date of sowing	Area in Bigha	Seed Qty. in Kg	Date of sowing	Area in Bigha	Seed Qty. in Kg	Date of sowing	Area in Bigha	Seed Qty. in Kg	Date of sowing	Area in Bigha	Seed Qty. in Kg	Date of sowing	Area in Bigha	Seed Qty. in Kg	Date of sowing	Area in Bigha	Seed Qty. in Kg	Date of sowing	Area in Bigha
1.	Sh. Dharam Pal Singh S/O Shri Raghuveer Singh	–	–	–	0.75	27.7.05	3 Bigha	–	–	–	50	8.9.05	5	–	–	–	–	–	–	–	–	–
2.	Sh. Ramveer Singh S/O Sri Atar Singh	4	26.7.05	5	0.75	27.7.05	3 Bigha	–	–	–	50	8.9.05	5	–	–	–	–	–	–	–	–	–
3.	Sh. Sardar Singh S/O Sh. Mangal Singh	1	1.8.05	1.25	–	–	–	0.500	24.7.05	1	–	–	–	–	–	–	0.500	24.7.05	2	–	–	–
4.	Sh. Rajpal Singh S/O Sh. Dhan Singh	1	1.8.05	1	0.75	1.7.05	1.50	0.250	1.8.05	0.5	50	8.9.05	50 plants	–	–	–	–	–	–	–	–	–
5.	Sh. Dinesh Kumar Singh S/O Sri Ram Singh	1	26.7.05	1	0.75	1.8.05	1.50	–	–	–	50	7.9.05	5	–	–	–	–	–	–	–	–	–
6.	Sh. Ashok Kumar Sharma S/O Om Prakash Sharma	1	24.7.05	1.25	–	–	–	–	–	–	–	–	–	–	–	–	0.500	25.7.05	2	–	–	–
7.	Sh. Pinku Singh S/O Sh. Panna Singh	1	24.7.05	1	0.75	24.7.05	1.50	–	–	–	–	–	–	–	–	–	–	–	–	–	–	–
8.	Sh. Sushil Babu Sharma S/O Sh. Chandra Pal Sharma	1	3.8.05	1.50	–	–	–	0.250	3.8.05	0.25	–	–	–	–	–	–	–	–	–	0.500	3.8.05	50 Plants
9.	Sh. Ram Prakash Chauhan S/O Sri Nahar Singh Chauhan	1	3.8.05	1.25	–	–	–	–	–	–	–	–	–	–	–	–	–	–	–	–	–	–
10.	Sh. Hari Om Chauhan S/O Sh. Nahar Singh Chauhan	1	3.8.05	1.25	–	–	–	–	–	–	–	–	–	–	–	–	–	–	–	–	–	–
11.	Sh. Brijendra Singh S/O Hazan Singh	1	3.8.05	1	–	–	–	–	–	–	–	–	–	–	–	–	–	–	–	0.500	3.8.05	50 Plants
12.	Sh. Shyam Veer Singh S/O Sh. Atar Singh	1	3.8.05	1.25	–	–	–	–	–	–	–	–	–	–	–	–	–	–	–	–	–	–
13.	Sh. Nam Pal Singh S/O Sh.Samsher Singh	1	24.7.05	1	–	–	–	–	–	–	–	–	–	–	–	–	–	–	–	–	–	–

SNO	Name of Farmer with Father's Name and Address	Ashwagandha(*Withania somnifera*),			Kalmegh(*Andrographis paniculata*)			Kaunch (*Mucuna pruriens*)			Bael Tree (*Aegle marmelos*)			Amla Tree (*Emblica officinalis*)			Kanta Karanj (*Caesalpinia bonduc* (L.) Roxb.			Jatropha (*Jatropha curcas*)		
		Seed Qty. in Kg	Date of sowing	Area in Bigha	Seed Qty. in Kg	Date of sowing	Area in Bigha	Seed Qty. in Kg	Date of sowing	Area in Bigha	Seed Qty. in Kg	Date of sowing	Area in Bigha	Seed Qty. in Kg	Date of sowing	Area in Bigha	Seed Qty. in Kg	Date of sowing	Area in Bigha	Seed Qty. in Kg	Date of sowing	Area in Bigha
14.	Sh. Pardeep Kumar Singh S/O Sh. Rajendra Singh	1	28.7.05	1	–	–	–	–	–	–	–	–	–	–	–	–	0.500	28.7.05	2	–	–	–
15.	Sh. Ashok Kumar Singh S/O Sh. Rajendra Singh	1	28.7.05	1	–	–	–	–	–	–	–	–	–	–	–	–	–	–	–	–	–	–
16.	Sh. Birendra Singh S/O Sh. Laxman Singh	3	31.7.05	3.5	–	–	–	–	–	–	–	–	–	–	–	–	–	–	–	–	–	–
17.	Sh. Surendra Singh S/O Sh. Laxman Singh	2	31.7.05	2.5	–	–	–	–	–	–	–	–	–	–	–	–	–	–	–	–	–	–
18.	Sh. Krishna Dutt Singh S/O Sh. Gajraj Singh	1	28.7.05	1	0.75	31.7.05	1.50	–	–	–	–	–	–	–	–	–	–	–	–	–	–	–
19.	Sh. Churaman Singh S/O Sh. Rohtas Singh	2	31.7.05	2.5	0.75	31.7.05	1.50	1	1.8.05	1	–	–	–	–	–	–	0.500	1.8.05	2.00	–	–	–
20.	Sh. Ashok Kumar Singh S/O Sh.Churaman Singh	1	31.7.05	1.5	0.75	31.7.05	1.50	–	–	–	–	–	–	–	–	–	–	–	–	–	–	–
21.	Sh. Amit Kumar Singh S/O Sh. Churaman Singh	1	31.7.05	1.5	0.75	31.7.05	1.50	–	–	–	–	–	–	–	–	–	–	–	–	–	–	–
22.	Sh. Yudhisthir Singh S/O Sh. Dharam Pal Singh	1	27.7.05	1.50	–	–	–	–	–	–	–	–	–	–	–	–	–	–	–	–	–	–
23.	Jitendra Singh S/O Sh. Samsher Singh	1	–	–	0.75	–	–	–	–	–	–	–	–	–	–	–	–	–	–	–	–	–
24.	Sh. Sudhir Kumar Singh S/O Sh. Dalveer Singh	1	27.7.05	1.50	–	–	–	–	–	–	–	–	–	–	–	–	–	–	–	–	–	–
25	Sh. Ram Kumar Singh S/O Sh. Lakhan Singh	2	31.7.05	2.50	–	–	–	–	–	–	50	9.8.05	5	–	–	–	–	–	–	–	–	–
26.	Sh. Ramesh Chandra Sharma S/O Sh. Bahori Lal Singh	–	–	–	–	–	–	–	–	–	50	6.8.05	5	–	–	–	–	–	–	–	–	–
27.	Sh. Manveer Singh S/O Sh. Panna Singh	–	–	–	–	–	–	–	–	–	50	8.9.05	5	–	–	–	–	–	–	–	–	–

SNO	Name of Farmer with Father's Name and Address	Ashwagandha(*Withania somnifera*),			Kalmegh(*Andrographis paniculata*)			Kaunch (*Mucuna pruriens*)			Bael Tree (*Aegle marmelos*)			Amla Tree (*Emblica officinalis*)			Kanta Karanj (*Caesalpinia bonduc* (L.) Roxb.			Jatropha (*Jatropha curcas*)		
		Seed Qty. in Kg	Date of sowing	Area in Bigha	Seed Qty. in Kg	Date of sowing	Area in Bigha	Seed Qty. in Kg	Date of sowing	Area in Bigha	Seed Qty. in Kg	Date of sowing	Area in Bigha	Seed Qty. in Kg	Date of sowing	Area in Bigha	Seed Qty. in Kg	Date of sowing	Area in Bigha	Seed Qty. in Kg	Date of sowing	Area in Bigha
28.	Sh. Shyam Babu Singh S/O Sh. Sardar Singh	–	–	–	–	–	–	–	–	–	50	8.9.05	5	–	–	–	–	–	–	–	–	–
29.	Sh. Om Veer Singh S/O Sh. Babulal Sharma	2	20.7.05	3	–	–	–	–	–	–	–	–	–	–	–	–	–	–	–	–	–	–
30.	Sh. Kishori Lal Jatav S/O Sh. Garib Das	2	20.7.05	3	0.75	27.7.05	1.50	–	–	–	–	–	–	–	–	–	–	–	–	–	–	–
31.	Sh. Ram Prasad Verma S/O Sh. Gajraj Singh; Bhutpura P.O. Talimnagar, Aligarh	2	30.7.05	2.50	0.75	–	1.50	–	–	–	50	5.8.05	4	–	–	–	–	–	–	–	–	–
32.	Sh. Soran Singh S/O Sh. Umarao Singh Vill. Bhutpura P.O. Talimnagar, Aligarh	2	26.7.05	2.50	0.100	26.7.05	2.50	–	–	–	50	5.8.05	4	40	5.8.05	4	–	–	–	–	–	–
33.	Sh. Sahab Singh S/O Sh. Sri Ram Singh Vill. Bhutpura P.O. Talimnagar, Aligarh	–	–	–	–	–	–	–	–	–	50	5.8.05	4	–	–	–	–	–	–	–	–	–
34.	Sh. Vijendra Singh S/O Sh. Hazari Lal	1	30.7.05	1.00	–	–	–	–	–	–	–	–	–	–	–	–	–	–	–	–	–	–
35	Sh. Than Singh S/O Sh. Mahaveer Singh	1	26.7.05	1.25	–	–	–	–	–	–	50	5.8.05	4	–	–	–	–	–	–	–	–	–
	Total	**42 Kg**		**81.250**	**1Kg**		**22.00**	**2.00**	**3Kg.**	**1 Bigha**	**610**		**56 Bigha**	**90**		**9 Bigha**	**2.00 Kg.**	—	**8 Bigha**	**1Kg**		**1 Bigha**

SNO	Name of Farmer with Father's Name	Sanai (*Cassia angustifolia*),			Safed Musli (*Chlorophytum borivilianum*)		
		Seed Qty. in Kg	Date of sowing	Area in Bigha	Seed Qty. in Kg	Date of showing	Area in Bigha
8	Sh. Sushil Babu Sharma S/O Sh. Chandra Pal Sharma	1	3.8.05	1.50	–	–	–
36	Dr. B. K. Singh S/O Sri Gajraj Singh	–	–	–	50	30.7.05	6.00

APPENDIX II

DETAILS OF SOME 53 FARMERS OUT OF 150 WESTERN U.P. FARMERS CULTIVATING MEDICINAL CROPS IN AN AREA OF 0.5-1 HECTARE DURING 2022-23.

SNO	Name farmer	Village	District	Crop
1	Dhyanpal Singh	Panihawar	Aligarh	Ashwagandha
2	Ganendra Pal Singh	Panihawar	Aligarh	Satawar
3	Munni Devi	Panihawar	Aligarh	Satawar
4	Nepal Singh	Panihawar	Aligarh	Ashwagandha
5	Krishna Pal Singh	Panihawar	Aligarh	Ashwagandha
6	Ramesh Pal Singh	Panihawar	Aligarh	Ashwagandha
7	Ashutosh	Mukatpur	Aligarh	Ashwagandha
8	Pramod Kumar	Potha	Aligarh	Ashwagandha
9	Akhilesh	Meerpur	Bulandshahr	Muskdana, Jatropha
10	Nem Singh	Natha Nagala	Aligarh	Ashwagandha
11	Umesh Kumar	Potha	Aligarh	Ashwagandha
12	Har Prasad	Nehraula (Khair)	Aligarh	Ashwagandha
13	Ashok Kumar	Rustampur Dhanipur	Aligarh	Satawar

SNO	Name farmer	Village	District	Crop
14	Buddhpal Singh	Panihawar	Aligarh	Ashwagandha
15	Vimlesh Kumar	Panihawar	Aligarh	Satawar
16	Ranjeet Singh	Gorna Rasidpur	Aligarh	Ashwagandha
17	Shyoraj Singh	Bhupal Nagariya	Aligarh	Ashwagandha
18	Durjan Singh Tomar	Saharanpur Godha	Aligarh	Tulsi
19	Chhatrapal Singh	Nagariya Pala Sallu	Aligarh	Tulsi
20	Nathi Singh	Pairal	Aligarh	Satawar
21	Dharmendra Singh	Gonda	Aligarh	Satawar
22	Rajesh Kumar Paliwal	Amritpur	Aligarh	Satawar
23	Om Prakash	Chandaus	Aligarh	Satawar
24	Sandeep Kumar	Jauhra Chandaus	Aligarh	Haldi, Tulsi
25	Onkar Singh	Machar	Bulandshahr	Satawar
26	Prempal Singh	DanukaTappal	Aligarh	Kalmegh
27	Hakim Singh	Salpur	Aligarh	Ashwagandha
28	Prempal Singh	Nagariya Jalesar Road	Hathras	Kalmegh, Satawar, Tulsi
29	Rajveer Singh	Shahjadpur	Hathras	Satawar
30	Ramveer Singh	Padu Mursang	Hathras	Satawar, Ashwagandha
31	Suneel Kumar Raghav	Mahmadpur	Bulandshahr	Ashwagandha
32	Subhash Chauhan	Kasimpur	Aligarh	Kalmegh, Haldi
33	Praduman	Shihora	Mathura	Ashwagandha
34	Anand Singh Chauhan	Talwar Dibai	Bulandshahr	Satawar
35	Ram Singh Chauhan	NOIDA	GB Nagar	Satawar, Tulsi, Ashwagandha

SNO	Name farmer	Village	District	Crop
36	Yogendra Pal Singh	Rajpur	Firozabad	Satawar
37	Rajveer Singh	Chendola Sujanpur	Aligarh	Tulsi
38	Mahendra Kumar Paliwal	Etah	Etah	Kalmegh, Tulsi
39	Om Prakash	Foji Baldev	Mathura	Ashwagandha
40	Ram Kishan	Ramgarh	Etah	Ashwagandha
41	Jain Degree College	Bahjoi	Sambal	Ashwagandha, Satawar
42	Sudhir Sukla	Sahpau	Hathras	Ashwagandha
43	Gajendra Pal Singh	Suhawali	Aligarh	Ashwagandha
44	Mahipal Singh	Kochod Balipur	Aligarh	Ashwagandha
45	Rajendra Singh	Bhojraj	Aligarh	Ashwagandha
46	Kishan Pal Singh	Madhu Ka Nagala	Hathras	Ashwagandha
47	Dushyant Kumar	Dhoodhama	Aligarh	Kalmegh
48	Durjan Singh	Saharanpur, Gonda	Aligarh	Tulsi
49	Jubbhan Singh	Saharanpur, Gonda	Aligarh	Tulsi
50	Ratan Singh	Saharanpur, Gonda	Aligarh	Tulsi
51	Veerendra Singh	Vrindavan	Mathura	Tulsi
52	Chhatra Shal	Mohatipur	Bulandshahr	Satawar
53	Narendra Kumar Tiyagi	Hapur	Hapur	Satawar

APPENDIX III

LIST OF MEDICINAL PLANTS CURRENTLY SUPPORTED FOR CULTIVATION BY THE NATIONAL MEDICINAL PLANTS BOARD, GOVERNMENT OF INDIA, NEW DELHI:

S. No.	Botanical Name	Common Name
1	*Abies webbiana Lindl*	Talispatra
2	*Abrus precatorius* L.	Chirmati,Chinnoti,
3	*Acacia catechu* Willd	Katha
4	*Aconitum chasmanthum* Stapf	Vatsnabh(API)
5	*Aconitum ferox Wall./A. balfouri*	Vatsnabh
6	*Aconitum heterophyllum* Wall.exRoyle	Atees
7	*Acorus calamus* Linn.	Vach
8	*Adhatoda zeylanica*	Adusa
9	*Aegle marmelos* (Linn) Corr.	Beal
10	*Albizzia lebbeck* Benth.	Shirish
11	*Aloe vera* (Linn.)Burn.	Ghritkumari
12	*Alpinia calcarata* (Haw.) Ros.	Smaller Galangal
13	*Alpinia galangal* (L.)Willd.	GreaterGalanga
14	*Alstonia scholaris* R.Br.	Satvin,Saptaparna
15	*Altingia excelsa* Noronha	Silarasa
16	*Anacyclus pyrethrum* DC.	Akarkara
17	*Andrographis paniculata* (Linn.) Burn	Kalmegh

S. No.	Botanical Name	Common Name
18	*Aquilaria agallocha* Roxb.	Agar
19	*Artemisia annua* (Linn.)	Artemisia
20	*Asparagus racemosus* Willd.	Shatavari
21	*Atropa belledona* L.	Atropa
22	*Azadirachta indica* A.Juss	Neem
23	*Bacopa monnieri* (L.) Pennell	Brahmi
24	*Berberis aristata* DC.	Daruhaldi
25	*Bergenia ciliate* Stern.	Pashnabheda
26	*Boerhaavia diffusa* Linn.	Punarnava
27	*Caesalpinia sappan* Linn.	Patang
28	*Cassia angustifolia* Vahl.	Senna
29	*Catharanthus roseus* (L.) G. Don.	Sadabahar
30	*Celastrus paniculatus*	Malkangani,Jyothismathi,BavanthiBeeja
31	*Centella asiatica* (Linn.)Urban	Mandookparni
32	*Chlorophytum borivillianum* Sant.	ShwetMusali
33	*Cinnamomum tamala* (Buch-Ham) Nees	Tezpatta
34	*Cinnamomum verum* Presl	Dalchini
35	*Cinnamomum camphora*	Kapoor
36	*Clerodendrum phlomoidis* L.f	Arni
37	*Clitoria ternatea* L.(Blue & White veriety)	Aparajita
38	*Coleus barbatus* Benth.Syn. Coleus forskholii	PatherChur
39	*Coleus vettiveroides* K.C.Jacob	Hrivera
40	*Commiphora wightii* (Arn.) Bhandari	Guggal
41	*Convolvulus microphyllus*	Shankhpushpi
42	*Coptisteeta Wall.*	Mamira
43	*Coscinum fenastratum* (Gertn) Colebr.	PeelaChandan
44	*Crataeva nurvala* Buch–Ham.	Varun
45	*Cryptolepis buchanani* Roem & schult	Krsnasariva
46	*Curculigo orchioides*	KaliMusali,Muslishiya
47	*Curcuma augustifolia*	Tikhur
48	*Dacalophis hamiltonii*	Nannari
49	*Dactylorhiza hatagirea hatagirea* (D.Don)	Salampanja

S. No.	Botanical Name	Common Name
50	*Desmodium gangeticum*	Sarivan
51	*Digitalis purpurea* Linn.	Foxglove
52	*Dioscorea bulbifera* Linn.	Rotalu,Gethi
53	*Eclipta alba* Hassk.	Kesuria,Bhangra,Ajagara,Bringaraj
54	*Embelia ribes* Burm. f.	Vai Vidang
55	*Emblica officinalis* Gaertn.	Amla
56	*Ephedra gerardiana* ***Wall.***	Somlata
57	*Ferula foetida* Regel.	Hing
58	*Garcinia indica* Choisy	Kokum
59	*Gentiana kurroo* Royle	Trayamana
60	*Ginkgo biloba*	Ginkgo
61	*Gloriosa superb* Linn.	Kalihari
62	*Glycyrrhiza glabra* Linn.	LicoriceRoots,Mulethi
63	*Gmelina arborea* Linn.	Gambhari
64	*Gymnema sylvestre* R.Br.	Gudmar
65	*Hedychium spicatum* Buch- Ham. exSmuth	Kapurkachari
66	*Hemidesmus indicus* R.Br.	Anantmool,IndianSarsaparilla
67	*Hippophae rhamnoides* Linn.	Seabuckthorn
68	*Holarrhena antidysenterica* Wall.	Kurchi/Kutaj
69	*Hyoscyamus niger* L.	Khurasaniajwane
70	*Inula racemosa* Hk.f.	Pushkarmool
71	*Ipomoea mauritiana/Ipomoea digitata*	Giantpotato
72	*Ipomoea petaloidea* Choisy	Vrddhadaruka
73	*Ipomoea turpethum* R.Br.	Trivrit
74	*Juniperus cumminis* Linn	Hapushal,Hanber,Bethar,Hapusha
75	*Jurineana crocephala* Benth.	Dhoop,Jari-dhoop
76	*Kaempferia galanga* L.	Indiancrocus
77	*Lepidum sativum* Linn.	Chandrasur
78	*Leptadenia reticulate* (Retz)Wt.&Arn.	Jivanti
79	*Litsea glutinosa* (Lour.) Robinson	Listea
80	*Mappia foetida* Miers.	Ghanera
81	*Mesua ferrea* Linn.	Nagakeshar
82	*Moringa olifera* Lamk.	Sahjan
83	*Mucuna prurita* Linn.	Konch
84	*Nardostachys jatamansi* DC.	Jatamansi

S. No.	Botanical Name	Common Name
85	*Ocimum sanctum* Linn.	Tulsi
86	*Onosma hispidum* Wall. ex Don	Ratanjot
87	*Oroxylum indicum* Vent.	Syonaka
88	*Panax pseudo-ginseng* Wall	Ginseng
89	*Phyllanthus amarus* Schum & Thonn.	Bhumi amlaki
90	*Picrorhiza kurroa* Benth. Ex Royle	Kutki
91	*Piper cubeba* Linn. f.	Kababchini
92	*Piper longum* Linn.	Pippali
93	*Plantago ovate* Forsk.	Isabgol
94	*Pluchea lanceolata* (DC)CB Clark.	Rasna
95	*Plumbago rosea* (L.)	Leadwort
96	*Plumbago zeylanica* Linn.	Chitrak
97	*Podophyllum hexandrum* Royle.	Bankakri,Indianpodophyllum
98	*Polygonatum cirrhifolium* Wall.	Mahameda
99	*Premna integrifolia* Linn.	Agnimanth
100	*Pseudarthria viscid* (L.) Wt & Arh	Moovila
101	*Psoralea corylifolia* L.	Bakuchi
102	*Pterocarpus marsupium* Roxb.	Beejasar
103	*Pterocarpus santalinus* Roxb.	Raktachandan,Redsanders
104	*Pueraria tuberose* DC.	Vidarikand
105	*Rauwolfia serpentine* Benth. Ex Kurz	Sarpgandha
106	*Rheum emodi* Wall ex Meissn	Archa
107	*Rubia cordifolia* Linn	Manjishtha
108	*Salacia reticulate* Wight	Saptachakra(Saptarangi)
109	*Santalum album* Linn.	Chandan
110	*Saraca asoca* (Roxb.) De Wilde	Ashok
111	*Saussurea costus* C.B. Clarke	Kuth,Kustha
112	*Sida cordifolia* (L.)	Flannelweed
113	*Smilax china* Linn.	Hrddhatri(Madhusnuhi), Lokhandi
114	*Solanum anguivi* Lamk	Katheli-badhi
115	*Solanum nigrum* Linn.	Makoy
116	*Stereospermum suaveolens* DC.	Patala
117	*Stevia rebaudiana* (Bert.) Hem.	Madhukari
118	*Swertia chirata* Buch-Ham	Chirata,Charayatah
119	*Symplocos racemosa* Roxb	Lodh/Pathani
120	*Tacomella undulate* (Sm.) Seem.	Rohitak

S. No.	Botanical Name	Common Name
121	*Taxus wallichiana* Linn.	Thuner,Talispatra
122	*Tephrosia purpurea* Pers	Pawad,Sharapunkha,
123	*Terminalia arjuna* (Roxb.)Wt.&Arn.	Arjuna
124	*Terminalia bellirica* Gaertn.	Behera
125	*Terminalia chebula* Retz.	Harad
126	*Tinospora cordifolia* Miers	Giloe
127	*Tragia involucrate* (L.)	Barhanta
128	*Trichosanthes cucumerina* (L.)	Patolpanchang
129	*Tricopus zeylanicus* Gartner	Jeevani
130	*Tylophora asthmetica* Wt & Arn.	Damabooti
131	*Urarea picta* (Jacq.) Desv.	Prishnaparni
132	*Valeriana hardwickii* (Wall) Wight	Tagar-ganth,Nihani
133	*Valerian awallichi* DC.	IndianValerian
134	*Vateria indica* (L.)	Mandadhupa,Dupa
135	*Vetiveria zizanoides* (L.) Nash	Khas-khasgrass
136	*Viola odorata* L.	Bunafsha
137	*Vitex nigundo* (L.)	Nirgundi
138	*Withania somnifera* (Linn.)Dunal	Ashwagandha
139	*Woodfordia fruticosa Kurz.*	Dhataki
140	*Zanthoxylum alatum* (Roxb.) Roxb.	Timoor

Source: Personal communication, National Medicinal Plants Board, Government of India, New Delhi.

APPENDIX IV

AGROTECHNIQUES OF SELECTED MEDICINAL CROPS RECOMMENDED FOR COMMERCIAL CULTIVATION HAVING ASSURED MARKET

In the context of global trade practices, it is essential to cultivate superior varieties of medicinal crops that possess the required active constituents to command higher prices and gain early acceptance from buyers. This necessitates proper identification and standardization of medicinal crops to ensure the safety and quality of raw produce.

The appendix presents agro-techniques and cost-benefit ratios of select medicinal crops, based on the personal field experience of the author. These species are well-suited to the agro-climatic conditions of Western Uttar Pradesh and were successfully cultivated by farmers during the period 2002 to 2006.

Cultivation Practices of Key Medicinal Crops Recommended to Farmers

S. No.	Common Name	Botanical Name
1	Amla	*Emblica officinalis* Gaertn
2	Ashwagandha	*Withania somnifera*
3	Bael	*Aegle marmelos* (L.) Corr.
4	Isabgol	*Plantago ovata* Forsk
5	Kalmegh	*Andrographis paniculata* Nees

S. No.	Common Name	Botanical Name
6	Safed Musli	*Chlorophytum (borivilianum)* Sant.
7	Senna	*Cassia angustifolia* Vahl.
8	Shatavari	*Asparagus racemosus* Willd.
9	Tulsi	*Ocimum sanctum* Linn.
10	Kanta Karanj	*Caesalpinia bonducella* (L.) Fleming
11	Kasni	*Cichorium intybus* Linn.

Precautions Before Undertaking Cultivation of Medicinal Crops:

पश्चिमी उत्तर प्रदेश में औषधीय पादपों के विषय में जागरूकता अभियान एवं खेती कि परियोजना

(राष्ट्रीय औषधीय पादप बोर्ड, भारत सरकार, नई दिल्ली द्वारा अनुदानित)

खेती प्रारम्भ करने से पहले उपयोगी जानकारी

1. जड़ी बूटी की खेती से सम्बंधित साहित्य जो उपलब्ध हो सके, प्राप्त कर ले।
2. जहाँ भी सफल खेती हो रही है, उसका अवलोकन करें तथा अनुभवों का लाभ उठायें। कृषिकरण, पादप के औषधीय भागों का संग्रह का तरीका विपणन कि जानकारी प्राप्त कर लें।
3. खेती शुरू करने से पहले अपनी क्षमता का मूल्यांकन कर लें। खेती आप स्वयं करेंगे या करायेंगे। जमीन की प्रकार, उपज की स्थिति, सिंचाई, निराई, खाद आदि की उचित व्यवस्था जलवायु तथा आर्थिक स्थिति का आंकलन कर लें।
4. आपके उत्पाद की खपत कहाँ और कैसे होनी है। उसकी उचित व्यवस्था कर लें।
5. आप जिस जड़ी बूटी की खेतीकर रहे है, वह बाजार में किस रूप में बिकती है – जड़, तना, छाल, पत्ती, बीज, फूल अथवा पंचांग।
6. अपने क्षेत्र में उगने योग्य 4-5 तरह के औषधीय पौधों को प्रयोगात्मक रूप से उगाये। सिमित या उपलब्ध साधनों में जिसकी उपज अच्छी हो उसे आगे के लिए चुने तथा बड़े भाग में खेती करें।
7. जहाँ तक हो अच्छा बीज /प्लांटिंग भाग प्राप्त करें। अभी ज्यादातर खेती योग्य पौधों के बीजों का प्रमाणीकरणनहीं हो पाया है। अतः अच्छा बीज प्राप्त कर स्वयं अपनी आवश्यकताके लिए बीज /प्लांटिंग भाग तैयार करें। उत्तम बीज उत्पादन कि जानकारी व तरीका आपको बताया जा सकता है।
8. जैविक खाद का प्रयोग करें। रसायनिक खाद का प्रयोग न करें।
9. ज्यादातर औषधीय पौधों में बीमारी नहीं होती। उपचारसे जयादा बचाव पर ध्यान दें। (प्राकृतिक तरीके से)
10. एक या दो फसल उगाकर अपनी पहचान बनायें। |

डा. वी. के. सिंह
परियोजना निदेशक

1. Amla (*Emblica officinalis* Gaertn.)

Common Names: Amlaki, Indian Gooseberry, Aonla, Amlika

Part Used

Fruit

Cultivation Practices

Soil and Climate

Amla thrives in a wide range of soils, except for pure sandy soils. Calcareous soils with a rocky sub-stratum are also suitable. For optimum yield, rich, loamy, well-drained soils are preferred. The plant can tolerate moderately alkaline and arid conditions. It grows well in tropical climates and performs satisfactorily with annual rainfall between 630–800 mm. Young plants under three years of age should be protected from frost in winter and hot winds in May and June. Mature trees can withstand temperatures as high as 46°C and even occasional sub-zero conditions.

Propagation and Planting

Although amla is commonly propagated by seed, seed-grown trees have a long juvenile phase and produce inferior-quality fruits. Shield budding on one-year-old seedlings using scions from high-yielding, superior mother plants is preferred. Even old, low-performing trees can be rejuvenated through top-working.

Pits of 1 meter^3 should be dug in May and June at 4.5-meter spacing and left open to sunlight for 15–20 days. Before planting, the topsoil should be mixed with 15 kg of well-rotted farmyard manure (FYM) and 1 kg of superphosphate.

Weeding and Hoeing

Weeding and hoeing are essential during the early growth phase, especially in nurseries.

Manures and Fertilizers

In addition to the initial 15 kg of FYM, young plants should receive 15–20 kg of FYM annually (September–October). Mature trees require 30–40 kg of FYM annually. Manure and Fertilizers should include:

- 30 grams of nitrogen annually during the early years (Sept–Oct).
- For mature trees, an annual dose of:
  - 1 kg Urea
  - 1 kg Superphosphate
  - 1.5 kg MOP

    This should be applied in two equal splits: once in September–October and again in April–May after fruit setting. Water the trees immediately after Fertilizers.

Irrigation

Amla requires minimal irrigation during the monsoon. During summer, young plants should be watered every 15 days until fully established. Fruit-bearing trees benefit from irrigation every two weeks during summer to enhance fruit setting and minimize fruit drop. Drip irrigation is highly effective—providing 25–30 liters of water per tree per day from October to December ensures good yield.

Harvesting and Post-Harvest Handling

Seedling-grown trees begin fruiting in 7–8 years, while budded trees start in 4–5 years. The fruits turn from light green to a dull greenish-yellow as they ripen, with **February** being the ideal harvest time due to peak ascorbic acid levels. In South India, fruits are available year-round.

Since ripe fruits are firm and do not drop easily, harvesting requires mechanical agitation or picking with bamboo poles fitted with hooks. After harvest, fruits should be graded by size to improve market value.

Yield

- A well-maintained 10-year-old tree produces 50–70 kg of fruit annually.
- Each kg contains approximately 15–20 fruits.

- A single tree can remain productive for up to 70 years, with peak yields occurring between 10–50 years.

Economics

- Cost of establishment (per hectare): ₹34,000
- Annual yield (8-year-old plantation): 20–25 tons
- Market price: ₹30–45 per kg
- Net income per hectare: ₹20,000

2. Ashwagandha (*Withania somnifera* (Linn.) Dunal)

Common Names: Asgandh, Nagouri Asgandh, Punir

Parts Used

Root, leaf, and seed

Cultivation Practices

Soil and Climate

Ashwagandha performs best in light red or sandy loam soils with good drainage and a pH between 7.5 and 8.0. It can be cultivated at altitudes of 600–750 meters. The crop requires a dry growing season and is well-suited for semi-tropical regions receiving 500–750 mm of rainfall. Ideal temperatures for its growth range between 20°C and 35°C. Late winter rainfall supports healthy root development.

Land Preparation

Ashwagandha is often cultivated on lands unsuitable for food crops due to limited irrigation. The soil is finely tilled using a plough, disc, or harrow and then levelled. These lands can be utilized profitably for Ashwagandha cultivation due to the crop's low water and fertility demands.

Nursery Raising and Planting

The crop may be sown by broadcasting or in lines, with the line method preferred for better root development and easier intercultural operations. Seeds are sown 1–3 cm deep in June or July in nurseries.

A light shower after sowing promotes good germination. Approximately 500–750 grams of seed are sufficient for one hectare.

To prevent seed-borne diseases, seeds should be treated with Thiram, Indofil, or Dithane M-45 at 3 g/kg before sowing. After 25–35 days, seedlings can be transplanted to the field at 60×60 cm spacing. As a Kharif (rainy season) crop, sowing should align with the onset of the monsoon in the region.

Thinning and Weeding

To maintain a plant population of around 30–60 plants per square meter (approx. 3.5–6 lakh plants/hectare), manual thinning is done 25–30 days after sowing. Plant density varies with soil fertility and terrain. On marginal lands or with the use of NPK (20:20:0) fertilizer, lower density is advisable. Early hand weeding is sufficient, as mature Ashwagandha plants naturally suppress weed growth.

Manure and Fertilizers

Ashwagandha requires minimal Fertilizers. In commercial cultivation areas such as Madhya Pradesh, it is grown on residual soil fertility without added fertilizers. Research from the Indore Research Station indicates that nitrogen and phosphorus have little effect on root yield.

Irrigation

Ashwagandha generally does not require irrigation if rainfall is adequate. Light rain after transplanting helps seedlings establish. Over-irrigation or excessive rainfall can harm the crop. Emergency irrigation may be applied during dry spells if necessary.

Harvesting and Post-Harvest Handling

Flowering and fruiting begin in December, and the crop is ready for harvest 150–180 days after sowing, typically between January and March. Maturity is indicated by yellow-red berries and drying leaves. Plants are uprooted and the stems are cut 1–2 cm above the crown to separate roots from aerial parts.

Roots are either sun-dried whole or cut into transverse segments of 7–10 cm. Yield per acre is approximately 650–800 kg of fresh roots, which reduces to 350–435 kg after drying. Berries are hand-picked, dried, and crushed to extract seeds.

Further cleaning, trimming, and grading are necessary. Roots are gently beaten to remove adhering soil and lateral rootlets. Remaining stems, crowns, and side branches are trimmed with a knife.

Yield

On average, 3–5 quintals (300–500 kg) of dried roots and 50–75 kg of seeds can be harvested per hectare under commercial cultivation.

Economics

- Cost of cultivation per hectare: ₹5,600
- Gross return per hectare: ₹30,000
- Net income: ₹24,000

Note: The market for medicinal plants is volatile; actual returns may vary.

---

3. Bael (*Aegle marmelos* Correa ex Roxb.)

Common Names: Bilva, Holy Fruit Tree, Bel

Parts Used

Fruit, root, and leaves

Cultivation Practices

Soil and Climate

Bael thrives in warm, humid climates with good sunlight and sandy loam soils that offer proper drainage.

Nursery Raising and Planting

Propagation is typically by seed. Sowing is done in June or July, but seedlings grow slowly and must remain in the nursery for at least one year before transplanting. Transplantation is done during the rainy season when seedlings have developed 3–5 leaves and a taproot of 20–25 cm.

Vegetative propagation is also possible via root or stem cuttings treated with Indole-3-butyric acid (IBA) at 4000 ppm. In the field, seedlings or budded plants are spaced 10–12 meters apart. While seedlings bear fruit in 7–8 years, budded plants begin fruiting in 4–5 years.

Manure, Thinning, and Weeding

In the first year, the plants should be well-manured and weeded after the monsoon to promote strong early growth.

Irrigation

Irrigate the field weekly or biweekly after planting, depending on weather conditions and soil moisture.

Harvesting and Post-Harvest Handling

Fruits mature slowly, taking about a year to ripen. Initially green, they turn yellow upon ripening. Fruits are harvested with their stalks, which detach easily only when fully ripe.

Yield

Each mature tree can yield 300–400 fruits annually. The quality of fruits depends significantly on the size and weight of the seed sacs; larger, heavier sacs often have more mucilage, indicating inferior quality.

Economics

- Market price of fruit pulp: ₹40–₹45 per kg

---

4. Isabgol (*Plantago ovata* Forsk.)

Common Names:

Ishagola, Isabghul, Spogel Seed, Ispaghal.

Part Used:

Husk from spikes and seeds.

Cultivation:

Soil and Climate:

Isabgol prefers light, well-drained soil with a pH of 4.7 to 7.7. It requires irrigation and thrives in warm temperatures. Ideal sowing is in the first week of November for the highest yields. Avoid early sowing (downy mildew risk) and late sowing (seed shattering from summer rains). Best germination occurs at 20–30°C.

Land Preparation:

Clear the field of clods and weeds. Incorporate 10–15 tonnes of farmyard manure (FYM) per hectare during final ploughing. Divide the field into manageable plots, such as 8.0m x 3.0m.

Nursery and Planting:

Use fresh seeds from the previous crop for better germination. Treat seeds with a mercurial seed dresser to prevent damping-off. Mix seeds with fine sand or sieved manure before sowing. Scatter seeds evenly and lightly brush them with a broom to avoid deep burial. Irrigate immediately after sowing.

Weeding and Hoeing:

Regular hoeing and weeding are essential.

Fertilizers:

Apply 50 kg of nitrogen, 25 kg of P_2O_5, and 30 kg of K_2O (NPK) per hectare. Half the nitrogen and all phosphorus and potassium should be applied during sowing. The remaining nitrogen is applied a month later.

Irrigation:

Water lightly right after sowing. Germination starts in 6–7 days; if delayed, irrigate again. Additional irrigations are needed as the crop develops, with 6–7 total irrigations for optimal yield.

Harvesting and Post-Harvest:

The crop blooms 2 months after sowing and is ready for harvest in 110–130 days (February to March). Harvest when the plant is dry, after 10 AM, to avoid seed cracking. If spikes are compressed, seeds will fall out.

Yield:

- Gujarat Isabgol-1: 800–900 kg per hectare.
- Gujarat Isabgol-2: 1,000 kg per hectare.

Economics :

- Expenditure: Rs. 25,000 per hectare
- Return: Rs. 63,000 per hectare
- Net Income: Rs. 38,000

---

5. Kalmegh (*Andrographis paniculata* Wall. ex Nees)

Common Names:

Hara-Chiretta, Kalmegh

Part Used:

Whole plant

Cultivation:

Soil and Climate:

Kalmegh thrives in loamy to lateritic soils with moderate fertility. It needs heat, humidity, and sunlight, growing well with the monsoon. Flowering starts in September, lasting until December.

Nursery and Planting:

- Propagate via seeds or vegetative growth from nodes.
- Seeds take 5–6 months to sprout.
- Prepare three 10×2 m beds in May with organic manure.
- Soak seeds in composted soil and water frequently until seedlings appear (6–7 days).

- Transplant in June, spacing plants 30–45 cm apart. Water after planting.

Thinning and Weeding:

Hoe and weed once to establish the crop. Weeds won't be an issue once the crop is established.

Manure/Fertilizer:

- Apply 80 kg nitrogen and 40 kg P_2O_5 per hectare.
- Split nitrogen into two doses, 30–45 days apart.
- Use 3–6 tonnes of farmyard manure for the nursery.

Irrigation:

Monsoon rains are usually sufficient, but pre-monsoon irrigation (2–3 times) may be needed. Autumn irrigation has minimal effect on biomass yield.

Harvesting and Post-Harvest:

- Harvest at 90–100 days when flowering begins in September.
- Dry the plant in the shade and grind it into powder.

Yield:

3.5–4.0 tonnes of dried herb per hectare.

Economics

- Expenditure: Rs. 10,000 per hectare
- Return: Rs. 43,000 per hectare
- Net Income: Rs. 33,000 per hectare

6. Musali Safaid (*Chlorophytum borivilianum* Sant.)

Common Name:

Safaid Musli

Part Used:

Tuberous root

Cultivation:

Soil and Climate:

Grows well in rich, well-drained loamy to sandy loam soils with good organic content. Requires warm, humid weather and adequate soil moisture for vegetative growth and root development.

Nursery Raising and Planting:

- **By Seeds**:
  Seeds have sharp edges and dark color. Sprouting takes 12–16 days. Sow seeds in a well-prepared, manured seedbed in June. Maintain moisture during the early monsoon and transplant seedlings in Kharif season with 30×15 cm spacing. Seed propagation is less vigorous than vegetative propagation.

- **Vegetative Propagation**:
  Rootstocks sprout in May (occasionally as early as April). After 4–6 days of rain, seedlings emerge from the soil. Root bunches should be removed in May and replanted in the field. Even 1 cm long rootstocks can sprout new plants. Plant at 30×15 cm spacing on 15–20 cm high ridges. For one hectare, 250–300 kg of rootstocks are needed. Musli Safaid can be intercropped with maize.

Manure/Fertilizer:

Apply 10–15 tonnes of farmyard manure (FYM) per acre for optimal plant growth.

Irrigation:

Wait for rain before planting. If rain doesn't occur, irrigate immediately after planting. Additional irrigation may be required every 10–15 days once the soil moisture decreases.

Weeding:

One or two weeding-cum-hoeing operations are needed to keep the soil permeable and free of weeds.

Harvesting and Post-Harvest:

- The crop matures in about 90 days. The leaves turn yellow and dry out from the collar area.
- Harvest in September or October when the leaves are dry.
- Dig out the fleshy roots, wash, and spread the tubers to dry in the shade for 4–7 days to remove moisture.

Yield:

Varies based on conditions but typically requires good care to achieve optimal production.

Economics

- Expenditure: Rs. 9,25,000 per hectare
- Return: Rs. 1,62,000 per hectare
- Net Income: Rs. 7,00,000 per hectare

---

7. Senna (*Cassia angustifolia* Vahl.)

Common Names:

Sanai, Marknadi, Sonmukhi, Sana

Part Used:

Leaves and Pods

Cultivation:

Soil and Climate:

Senna thrives in red and alluvial loams, preferring soils with a pH of 7–8.5. It requires well-drained soil and is highly susceptible to flooding. Best grown in warm weather, it can be cultivated in winter (October-November) or early summer (February-March). Requires 25–40 cm of rainfall from June to October.

Land Preparation:

- Deep ploughing followed by two cross-ploughing operations, harrowing, and levelling.
- Leave soil exposed to the sun for 110–115 days to dry perennial weeds.
- Mix farmyard manure (FYM) during the final ploughing and install irrigation pipes.

Nursery Raising and Planting:

- **Seed Propagation**:
  Seeds have a hard coat. Soak for 10–12 hours for 100% germination. Sow seeds 1.5–2.5 cm deep at 30 cm intervals. Germination begins on day 3 and completes in 14 days.
  Treat seeds with 2.5 g/kg of Thiram, Captain, or Agroson G.N. to prevent seedling blight.

Thinning and Weeding:

- First weeding/hoeing: 25–30 days after sowing.
- Second weeding: 75–80 days.
- Third weeding: 110 days.
- Pre-emergent herbicide (Teeflan, 4 kg/hectare) can improve yield and anthraquinone content.

Manure/Fertilizer:

- Apply 10–15 tons of FYM per hectare.
- For better leaf and pod production, apply 80 kg P_2O_5 and K_2O per hectare.
- 50% nitrogen at seeding, remaining 50% 90 days later.

Irrigation:

- Senna can be grown under rainfed conditions but benefits from semi-irrigation.
- 5–8 mild irrigations are ideal; heavy irrigation can harm the crop.

Harvesting and Post-Harvest:

- First Picking: 5–90 days for sennosides in foliage.
- Second Picking: 90–100 days for leaves and pods.
- Third Picking: 130–150 days for full harvest.
- Dry leaves and pods by spreading them thinly in open fields or in well-ventilated drying sheds for 10–12 days. Alternatively, use mechanical drying at 40°C.

Yield:

- Irrigated Conditions: 15 quintals of dry leaves and 7 quintals of pods per hectare.
- Rainfed Conditions: 10 quintals of leaves and 4 quintals of pods per hectare.

Economics

- Expenditure: Rs. 7,000 per hectare
- Return: Rs. 37,500 per hectare
- Net Income: Rs. 30,500 per hectare

---

8. Shatavari (*Asparagus racemosus* Willd.)

Common Names: Satamuli, Satavar, Abhiru, Satavari

Part Used: Tuberous root

Soil and Climate:

Thrives in subtropical and sub-temperate climates up to 1,400 m. Grows well in medium black soils with a pH of 7–8.

Land Preparation:

- Plough soil to 20–30 cm depth.

- Harrow 2–3 times, remove weeds, level ground, and construct 40–45 cm wide ridges with 15–20 cm furrows for irrigation.

Nursery Raising and Planting:

- Seeds: Soak in raised beds by April, spaced 5 cm apart. Germination starts after the first monsoon rain (June). Transplant seedlings to ridges (60×60 cm) after reaching 45 cm height.
- Vegetative Propagation: Split the rhizomatous disc at the stem base, ensuring each part has 2–3 tuberous roots and 2+ buds. Cover with 1 cm soil and water. Sprouting occurs in 8–10 days.

Weeding:

- Two weedings during the wet months, and another 2–3 months later.

Irrigation:

- Twice in winter and once monthly in summer, after the rainy season ends.

Manure/Fertilizer:

- Use organic manure for best results. No specific NPK requirements.

Harvesting and Post-Harvest:

- Harvesting: After 40 months, harvest in winter.
- Post-harvest: Peel the roots using a sharp knife (can be tough if delayed). Soak in boiling water for 10 minutes, then peel. Slice into small pieces and dry in the shade.

Yield:

- Per Plant: 2607 g of fresh root.
- Per Hectare: 5–7 tons of dry root.

Economics

- Expenditure: Rs. 10,027 per hectare
- Return: Rs. 36,000 per hectare
- Net Income: Rs. 25,973 per hectare

9. Tulsi (*Ocimum sanctum* Linn.)

Common names: Holy Basil, Krishna Tulsi.

Part used: Leaf, whole plant, seed.

Cultivation:

Soil and Climate:

Thrives in a range of soil types. It grows well in soils that range from rich loam to poor laterite, saline and alkaline to somewhat acidic. Soil that drains well promotes healthier vegetative growth. A situation where there is too much water might lead to root rot and stunted growth.

Low oil content plants can be grown in partially shaded environments. It grows best in humid environments with a considerable amount of rainfall. It has been discovered that long days and high temperatures are beneficial for plant development and oil production. It can be grown in a topical and subtopical climate up to 900 metres above sea level.

Land preparation

After the land is fine-tuned, it is divided into manageable-sized irrigation patches. When preparing land, it is best to add 15 tonnes of farmyard manure per hectare and thoroughly mix it into the soil.

Nursery raising and planting

The third week of February is when the nursery can be elevated, and the middle of April is when transplanting usually begins. Seeds are used to reproduce the plant. Farmyard manure should be added to raised seed bags, measuring 15” by 4’9”. The bags should be carefully prepared and manured. To raise the seedlings for planting one hectare of land, 200–300 g of seeds are sufficient. In the nursery beds, the seed should be sown 2 cm below the surface. After 8 to 12 days for the seeds to germinate, the seedlings reach the 4-5 leaf stage and are prepared for transplantation in around 6 weeks. To get a high herbage and oil yield per hectare, the seedlings are transplanted at 40 × 40 cm and 40 × 50 cm.

Weeding and hoeing

One month after planting comes the first round of weeding, followed by another four weeks later. It is adequate to do one hoeing after two months after planting.

Manure/ Fertilizer

The best materials are compost, vermi compost, and organic manure. For this crop, the ideal fertilizer dosage is 60 kg P2O5 and 120 kg nitrogen per hectare.

Irrigation

The moisture content of the soil determines whether to irrigate. During the summer, three irrigations per month are required; during the rainy season, none are. It is sufficient to do 12 to 15 irrigations a year.

Harvesting/ Post-harvesting

When the crop reaches full bloom, it is harvested. After 90 to 95 days of planting, the first crop is received. After that, it can be harvested every 65 to 75 days. In order to get a decent oil output and quantity, harvesting is typically done on bright, sunny days. If there was rain the day before, it is not ideal to harvest the crop.

Yield

Per hectare, about 5 tonnes of fresh herbage can be harvested twice or three times a year.

Economics

Expenditure per hectare Rs. 1, 000/-

Return per hectare Rs. 5, 000-6,000/- ($2_{1/2\ months}$)

Net income Rs. 4,000/- to 5,000/-

10. Common Chicory (*Cichorium intybus* Linn.)

Common Names:

Common Chicory, Coffee Weed, Kasni

Soil and Climate:

Thrives in well-drained sandy soils with calcium content. Prefers soil temperatures around 21°C and grows well in cool, dry weather.

Propagation, Planting, Spacing, Watering:

- **Seeds**: Sown 3 mm deep in October–November in plains, or March–April in hills.
- **Germination**: 7–14 days.
- **Planting**: Seedlings are transplanted in sandy or calcareous soil in protected areas.
- **Spacing**: 1–2 ft between plants.
- **Watering**: Regular watering, with more during dry spells.

Harvesting:

Matures by late May; harvest, dry in shade or kiln, then thresh and winnow. The root is collected in broken pieces.

Production:

- **Seeds Required**: 1–1.5 kg per acre.
- **Plants per Acre**: 85,000.
- **Market Price**: Rs. 60 per kg (seeds), Rs. 40 per kg (roots).

Storage:

Clean and dry roots in shade, then store in airtight containers in a cool, dry place.

11. Karanjwa, Kanta Karanj *(Caesalpinia bonducella* (L.) Fleming)

Part Used: Leaves, seeds, and root.

Climate and Soil:

A xerophytic plant that thrives in dry, hot subtropical and tropical regions. Best grown in red loamy soils rich in humus with good drainage.

Propagation:

- Seeds: Collected in November–December, seeds mature 5–15 days post-flowering and take 3 months to mature (October–December).
- Raising Propagules: In April-May, treat seeds with H_2SO_4 (sulphuric acid) for 6 minutes, then wash and soak in 300 ppm GA_3 for 6 hours to promote rapid germination.
- Seed Rate: 600–800g per hectare.

Land Preparation:

- Pits: 45 × 45 × 45 cm spaced 4 m × 4 m.
- Fertilizer: Apply 6-8 kg of FYM and 100:50:75 g NPK per plant before planting.

Planting:

- Transplant 30-45-day-old seedlings at 4 m × 4 m spacing after the onset of monsoon rains.
- Irrigate immediately if no rain follows transplanting.
- For 1 hectare, 625 seedlings are needed.

Intercropping:

- Grown best as a single crop. Annuals can be intercropped in the first few years.

Irrigation:

- Light irrigation daily for the first 15 days post-transplanting, then weekly or fortnightly as required. Furrow irrigation is recommended.

Interculture and Maintenance:

- Apply 150:60:160 g NPK per plant in the second year, and 200:100:150 g NPK from the third year onwards.
- Weed manually and apply fertilizers every 4 months.
- Gap filling and staking of seedlings should occur 30 days after planting.

Harvesting:

Crop Maturity and Harvesting:

- Flowering: Begins 2–3 years after planting.
- Pods and Seeds: Pluck between October-November.
- Wood: Harvested 10-15 years after planting in October-November.

Chemical Constituents:

- Pod shells contain 4% tannins.
- Bark contains 1.8% tannins and aromatic compounds like brazilin, sappanchalcone, and ceasalpin.

Yield:

- Pods: 2000–2500 kg per hectare/year.
- Seeds: 200–250 kg dry seeds per hectare/year.
- Wood: Estimates unavailable.

Economics:

- Cost per Hectare: Rs. 7,500 approx.
- Market Demand: Over 100 MT/year (2006/07).

Note: Prices are volatile dependent on market fluctuations

Source: Cultivation Practices of Some Commercially Important Medicinal Plants (2002), National Medicinal Plants Board (NMPB), New Delhi, with technical inputs from Dr. V.K. Singh, Dr. K.V. Billore, and Dr. Rajat Rashmi, Research Officers at NMPB, acknowledged by the Secretary (ISM&H), Ministry of Health & Family Welfare, Government of India.

ABOUT THE AUTHOR

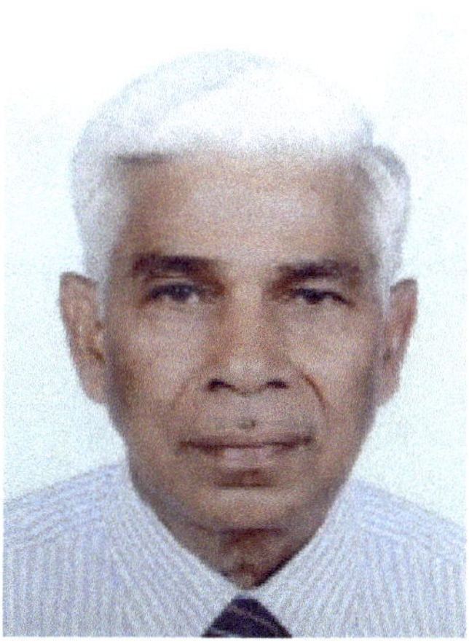

Dr. V.K. Singh is a plant taxonomist with a distinguished career in exploring medicinal plants, particularly in the realm of folk medicines and traditional knowledge. Through three decades of research in India's tribal-rich forest regions, he has documented a vast array of plant-based remedies. Dr. Singh's extensive publication record and numerous awards, including the Lifetime Achievement Award (2005), reflect his significant contributions to the field. He played a key role in promoting commercial medicinal crops cultivation nationwide during his tenure at the National Medicinal Plants Board, Government of India. Dr. V.K Singh concluded his career as Deputy Director (Botany) at CCRUM, Ministry of AYUSH, Government of India.

Email: vks_ccrum@yahoo.co.in

ABOUT THE BOOK

A pioneering work that presents a groundbreaking 'demonstration model' for promoting commercial medicinal crops cultivation among small-scale and marginal farmers in Western Uttar Pradesh, India. Drawing on the author's personal experience and a National Medicinal Plants Board-funded study, this book outlines a comprehensive approach to bridging the gap between awareness and full-fledged cultivation and marketing. Through documentation of agro-techniques, farmer meets, training sessions in vermicompost preparation, demonstration plots, and medicinal seed villages, this book offers practical insights and strategies for stakeholders. The book also discusses the present-day key challenges, opportunities, and strategies in India's medicinal farming sector. A valuable resource for new startups, Agri-entrepreneurs, government departments, and state medicinal plants boards across India, this work is poised to become a milestone in the evolving medicinal plants sector.